Nursing Documentation

made Incredibly Easy!®

Nursing Documentation

made
Incredibly
Easy!®

Fifth Edition

Clinical Editor
Kate Stout, RN, MSN
Post Anesthesia Care Staff Nurse
Grand Strand Memorial Hospital
Myrtle Beach, South Carolina

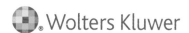 Wolters Kluwer

Philadelphia • Baltimore • New York • London
Buenos Aires • Hong Kong • Sydney • Tokyo

Executive Editor: Nicole Dernoski
Development Editor: Maria McAvey
Editorial Coordinator: Lindsay Ries
Production Project Manager: Linda Van Pelt
Design Coordinator: Elaine Kasmer
Manufacturing Coordinator: Kathleen Brown
Marketing Manager: Linda Wetmore
Prepress Vendor: Absolute Service, Inc.

5th edition

Copyright © 2019 Wolters Kluwer

9 8 7 6 5 4 3 2

Printed in China (or the United States of America)

Library of Congress Cataloging-in-Publication Data

Names: Stout, Kate, 1957- editor.
Title: Nursing documentation made incredibly easy! / clinical editor, Kate
  Stout.
Other titles: Charting made incredibly easy.
Description: Fifth edition. | Philadelphia : Wolters Kluwer, [2018] |
  Preceded by Charting made incredibly easy. 4th ed. c2010. | Includes
  bibliographical references and index.
Identifiers: LCCN 2018018484 | ISBN 9781496394736
Subjects: | MESH: Nursing Records | Documentation
Classification: LCC RT50 | NLM WY 100.5 | DDC 610.73--dc23 LC record available at
  https://lccn.loc.gov/2018018484

LWW.com

CCS0420

Dedication

To all the nurses who diligently document their patient assessments and care—you provide proof of what the profession does!

Kate Stout

Contributors

Cheryl L. Brady, RN, MSN
Assistant Professor
Kent State University
Salem, OH

Louise Colwill, RN, MSN
Medical-Surgical Clinical Nurse Specialist
MountainView Hospital
Las Vegas, NV

Laura Gartner, RN-BC, MSN
Senior Clinical Informatics Specialist
Abington Hospital–Jefferson Health
Abington, PA

Antoinette Pretto-Sparkuhl, RN, MSN
Chief Officer Quality, Safety, Value
Veterans Health Administration-VA
Southern Nevada Healthcare System

Marilyn D. Sellers, RN-BC, MS, FNP-BC
Family Nurse Practitioner
VA Medical Center
Hampton, VA

Donna Schultice, RN, MSN, FNP-BC, CEN
Staff Nurse—Emergency Department
Cooper University Hospital
Camden, NJ

Leigh Ann Trujillo, RN, BSN
Nurse Educator
St. James Hospital and Health Center
Olympia Fields, IL

Previous Contributors

Katrina D. Allen, RN, MSN, CCRN

Cheryl L. Brady, RN, MSN

Marie O. Brewer, RN, LNC

Roseanne Hanlon Rafter, RN, MSN, GCNS-BC

Joy L. Herzog, RN

Susan M. Kilroy, RN, MS

Donna Ratcliff, RN, MSN

Lauren R. Roach, LPN, HCS-D

Marilyn D. Sellers, RN-BC, MS, FNP-BC

Leigh Ann Trujillo, RN, BSN

Foreword

Providing the best care possible for your patients is the most important aspect of nursing. However, nurses find that documentation of that care can be very time consuming, taking time away from the bedside. Yet, documentation needs to be recognized as a crucial part of the health care system. Good nursing documentation clearly and concisely communicates the assessments, actions, and outcomes of care in a timely and accurate manner. Accurate documentation also plays a critical role in acquiring and maintaining accreditation for a facility. However, nurses continually struggle to document in a way that is timely, accurate, and legally prudent.

Although most facilities have converted to using an electronic health record, not all have had that opportunity, and paper documentation still exists. Examples are provided for a paper system because of the great variety in electronic systems and the complexity of utilizing those systems is too difficult to showcase by looking at one screenshot. However, the information presented throughout the book should be reflected in all documentation, whether on paper or electronic.

Nurses experience many barriers to completing documentation in an acceptable way. These include time, care complexity, and institutional policies associated with documentation. Whether you use paper or electronic charting, errors in documentation occur. Each type of documentation has errors specific to the type of documentation and there are errors common to all types of documentation. Learn your documentation system well in order to provide a record that meets professional and legal standards. Always remember, poor nursing documentation can place patients, staff, and organizations at considerable risk of physical and legal harm.

Kate Stout, RN, MSN
Post Anesthesia Care Staff Nurse
Grand Strand Memorial Hospital
Myrtle Beach, South Carolina

Contents

Chapter 1

Understanding documentation

Just the facts

In this chapter, you'll learn:
- ♦ the importance of documentation
- ♦ the components of a medical record
- ♦ types of medical records.

A look at documentation

Documentation is the process of creating a record of information. When associated with nursing, accurate, detailed documentation shows evidence of the extent and quality of the patient care you've provided, the outcome of that care, and treatment and education that the patient received, understood, and still needs.

Documentation is a vital communication tool among health care team members. Commonly, decisions, actions, and revisions related to the patient's plan of care are based on documentation from multidisciplinary team members. A well-documented medical record demonstrates a high degree of collaboration among health care team members.

You reach a wide audience

The information that's documented by health care team members must be easily retrievable, legible, and comprehensible because a patient's medical record may be read by a wide audience, including:
- other members of the health care team
- reviewers from accrediting, certifying, and licensing organizations
- performance-improvement monitors
- peer reviewers
- Medicare and insurance company reviewers
- researchers and teachers
- lawyers and judges.

One of the most compelling reasons for you to develop good documentation practices and skills is to provide proof that you've fulfilled your professional responsibility by meeting the standards of care.

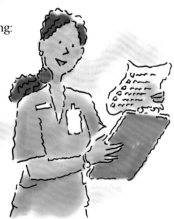

Wow! Great documentation! I can tell right away that the patient received thorough, high-quality care.

A short history of documentation

In the past, documentation consisted of cursory observations, such as *the patient ate well* or *the patient slept poorly*. The chief purpose of this type of documentation was to show that the practitioner's orders and the facility's policies had been followed and that the patient had received the proper care.

In the 19th century, the British nurse Florence Nightingale paved the way for modern nursing documentation. In the book, *Notes on Nursing*, she stressed the importance of training nurses to gather patient information in a clear, concise, organized manner. As her theories gained acceptance, nurses' perceptions and observations about patient care gained credence and respect. More than a century later, in the 1970s, nurses began creating their own vocabulary for documentation based on nursing diagnoses.

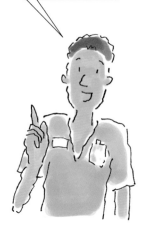

The history of documentation dates back to Florence Nightingale.

Role of documentation

Accurate nursing documentation is important for many reasons:
1. It provides communication among multidisciplinary care professionals.
2. It's used as a measure for evaluating appropriate actions.
3. It provides legal evidence that can protect you.
4. It aids research and education.
5. It assists facilities in obtaining and maintaining accreditation and licensure.
6. It justifies reimbursement requests.
7. It identifies the need for improvement in the quality or delivery of care.
8. It indicates compliance with the state nurse practice act.
9. It establishes professional accountability.

Communication

Patients are cared for by a multidisciplinary team, many of whom work different shifts. This creates an inability to speak directly with each other regarding the patient's condition or plan of care. The patient's medical record is the main source of information and communication among nurses, practitioners, respiratory and physical therapists, social workers, pharmacists, and other caregivers. Today, nurses are commonly considered managers of care as well as practitioners and usually document the most information. However, being able to access documentation of all health care team members presents a more complete picture of the patient's care, progress, and needs.

A growing team

As health care facilities continue to streamline and redesign care delivery systems, tasks that were historically performed by nurses now may be assigned to multiskilled workers. To deliver highly specialized care, each caregiver must provide accurate, thorough information and be able to interpret what others have documented to evaluate and plan future patient care.

Evaluation of actions

When health care is evaluated by administration, reviewers, insurance companies, Medicare representatives, lawyers, or judges, accurate nursing documentation is one way to prove that you're providing high-quality and accurate care. It's also a record of your patient's response to your care and any adjustments made to individualize the plan of care.

Legal protection

On the legal side, accurate documentation confirms that the care you provide meets the patient's needs and expressed wishes. It also proves that you're following the accepted standards of nursing care mandated by the law, your profession, and your health care facility.

The evidence speaks for itself

Accurate documentation communicates crucial clinical information to caregivers so they make fewer errors. How and what you document can determine whether you or your employer wins or loses a legal dispute. Medical records are used as evidence in cases involving disability, personal injury, death, and mental competency. Documentation is the pivotal issue in many malpractice cases.

Research and education

Documentation also provides data for research and continuing education. For example, researchers and nurse-educators may study medical records to determine the effectiveness of care or care systems. Their scrutiny may also reveal ways to improve documentation, such as by revising existing electronic documentation systems or creating specific forms for specialized documentation. The need for simple, accurate point-of-care documentation encourages researchers to develop new technologies to improve communication between health care providers, improve patient safety, and optimize a nurse's time.

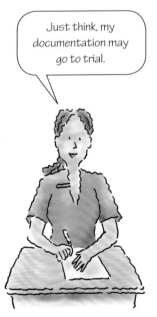

As nurses, we usually document the most information.

Just think, my documentation may go to trial.

A reciprocal relationship

Researchers also review individual medical records to gauge how patient teaching affects compliance and outcomes. As a result, they may identify the need for patient education materials or methods that are more effective.

Accreditation and licensure

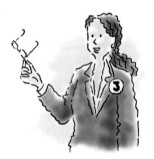

For a facility to obtain and maintain accreditation, caregivers must document care that reflects the standards set by national organizations, such as the Centers for Medicare & Medicaid Services and The Joint Commission. Some states also require facilities to be licensed; licensing laws, in turn, require each facility to establish policies and procedures for operation. (See chapter 6, Avoiding legal pitfalls, for more information.)

A facility's accreditation and licensure may be jeopardized by substandard documentation. Besides being complete and accurate, documentation must also be readable. (This requirement has driven many facilities to switch to an electronic health system.) When a facility is cited for having poor documentation or for not meeting set standards, a warning is given and a target date is set for the facility to make necessary changes and corrections. A facility may lose its license if these changes aren't accomplished.

Quality is key

In effect, accreditation is evidence that a facility provides quality care and is qualified to receive federal funds. The federal government works with state accrediting organizations to make sure facilities are eligible to receive Medicare reimbursement. Accreditation and reimbursement eligibility require documentation that accurately reflects the care provided to patients. Good documentation demonstrates that facility and state nursing policies have been followed.

Getting what they deserve

How do officials of accrediting organizations decide if a facility should be accredited? They look at the facility's structure and function. They also conduct surveys and audits of patient records and medical records to see if care meets the required standards.

Track with a tracer

To conduct their survey, The Joint Commission surveyors use an evaluation method called *tracer methodology*. They select a patient and use that patient's record to evaluate the organization's compliance with required standards. As part of the process, they interview the patient and caregivers about the care the patient received on this visit as well as previous visits. The patient's self-reports of care are then compared to nursing and other clinical documentation. Patient-reported care must match clinician-documented care.

Charting clinical competence

Furthermore, surveyors use the medical record to determine whether the patient received competent care from all clinicians, including nurses. During the evaluation process, the surveyor seeks to identify any performance or system level issues that affected patient care.

Is that safe?

Patient safety and medical errors are a national concern. The first National Patient Safety Goals (NPSGs) were approved by The Joint Commission in July 2002. Effective January 1, 2008, accredited hospitals must show that the NPSGs are implemented in daily care. The NPSGs are updated annually and can be found on The Joint Commission website.

Quality and consistency

Officials review charts and files to ensure good documentation. For example, in a case where physical restraints were used, officials may ask, "How is documentation completed regarding the need for restraints and their correct use?" and "Does the documentation in the charts show that restraints were used correctly?" Proper documentation reflects the quality of care provided and the facility's accountability.

Reimbursement

Reimbursement from Medicare and insurance companies depends heavily on accurate nursing documentation. For example, many hospitals today use elaborate electronic dispensing carts to keep track of supplies. Nursing documentation has to justify and register the use of these supplies to be reimbursed for them. Additionally, documentation of patient conditions and practitioner orders are reviewed to meet standards set by the federal government as best practice in order to receive annual funding or reimbursement. (See chapter 6, Avoiding legal pitfalls, for more information.)

It's payback time . . . or is it?

Documentation is also used to determine the amount of reimbursement a facility receives for care provided. The federal government, for example, uses a prospective payment system based on diagnosis-related groups (DRGs) to determine Medicare reimbursements. In other words, they pay a fixed amount for a particular diagnosis. For a facility to receive payment, the patient's medical record at discharge must contain the correct DRG codes and show that the patient received the proper care, including appropriate patient teaching and discharge planning.

Likewise, most insurance companies base reimbursements on a prospective payment system, and they usually don't reimburse for unskilled nursing care. They pay for skilled medical and nursing care only. For example, they compensate nurse practitioners and home health care nurses for skilled care, which includes assessing a patient's condition, creating a care plan, and following a strict treatment regimen.

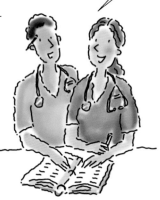

Your documentation also helps determine your facility's reimbursement.

Examinations aren't just for patients

Before reimbursing, an examiner studies the patient's medical record to decide whether the patient needed and received skilled nursing care. The examiner may request copies of the patient's monthly bills and look at documented progress notes, especially if the intensity, frequency, and cost of the care increased.

Examiners also check for inconsistencies in documentation, such as a discrepancy between the treatment ordered and the one provided. If the discrepancy isn't explained adequately, the insurer may deny payment.

Keeping the proper care going

In addition to keeping a facility from getting reimbursed, faulty documentation can keep patients from getting the care they need. For example, an insurer might deny payment to a home health care agency if the nurse's documentation doesn't prove that home visits were necessary. If that happens, home health care may be discontinued prematurely.

Performance improvement

Individual states and The Joint Commission require all health care facilities to regularly monitor, evaluate, and seek ways to improve the quality of care for their patients. In each facility, a committee of practitioners, nurses, pharmacists, administrators, and other employees meet to identify performance improvement needs. Committee members then implement improvement measures, analyze outcomes, and report their findings to the facility's board of trustees.

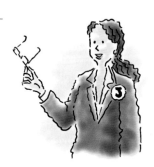

Multidisciplinary committee members also develop methods to assess the structure, process, and outcome of patient care. One way to implement these methods is to monitor and evaluate documentation.

Up to snuff?

What if the care described in a medical record doesn't meet an established standard? Performance improvement committee members look at the specific problem and create a plan to correct it. They may assign a focus group to investigate ways to do this.

The focus group may recommend changes in the facility's policies, procedures, or documentation forms in an effort to improve patient care. For example, many facilities have been cited in court for lack of documentation when physical restraints were used. As a result, some facilities have developed specific forms or computer screens to document restraint orders from practitioners, and care of the patient in restraints, which may be used in court as proof that the facility's policy was followed and that restraints were justified.

Nurse practice acts

Nurse practice acts are state laws that define what duties nurses can and can't perform in that specific state. State nurse practice acts are revised frequently; when nurse practice acts change, documentation requirements usually change as well. With laws and regulations in a constant state of flux, you must be especially meticulous about documentation of your care to show compliance with standards.

Accountability

Accurate nursing documentation is evidence that you acted as required or ordered. Accountability means you comply with the documentation requirements of your health care facility, professional organizations, and state law.

Types of medical records

Medical records are kept for virtually every person who steps through the door of a health care facility. That's a lot of documentation. This documentation may be completed using paper forms or electronically (or a combination of both) based on the specific facility. How can nurses deal with this responsibly and competently?

A comprehensive record

The medical record may be organized by category. However, this practice emphasizes form instead of content. Remember, a medical record isn't just a summary of illness and recovery. It's a record of a patient's personal information, health care wishes, practitioner's orders and evaluations, identified problems, diagnostic testing results, provided interventions, including administered medications, and

Tips for fast, faultless documentation

When you document, you must record information quickly without sacrificing accuracy. Here are some actions you can take to help you accomplish these two goals:
- Follow the nursing process.
- Use nursing diagnoses.
- Use flow sheets, if available.
- Document at the bedside.
- Individualize your documentation.
- Don't repeat information (which could lead to errors).
- Sign off with the date and time, your name, and credentials.
- Don't document for other caregivers.
- Use electronic systems, if available.

patient outcomes or response to interventions. (See *A close look at a medical record*, page 10.)

You can think of the medical record as an ally in your organization efforts. It's a place to organize your thoughts about patient care and record your actions. Used properly, it can help you save time, identify problem areas, plan better patient care, and avoid litigation. (See *Tips for fast, faultless documentation.*)

Although every medical record provides evidence of the quality of patient care, not all records are alike. Some are organized by a source-oriented narrative method, some by a problem-oriented method, and others by body system.

Source-oriented narrative method

With the source-oriented narrative method, caregivers (the source) from each discipline record information in a separate section of the medical record.

Missing the complete picture?

This traditional method of documentation has several serious drawbacks: Because documentation is done in various parts of the medical record, information is disjointed, topics aren't always clearly identified, and information may be difficult to retrieve. These issues may prevent team members from forming a complete picture of the patient's care and create breakdowns in communication.

Get on the same page

Collaboration among team members may be more successful if everyone documents in the same area. For example, practitioners', nurses', and respiratory therapists' progress notes can be combined into what may be called *patient progress notes*. These notes serve as the primary source of reference and communication among multidisciplinary health care team members.

Problem-oriented method

A problem-oriented medical record (POMR) is a centralized problem list that contains baseline data regarding a patient's medical needs. The problem list may contain acute and chronic conditions that may be related to providing appropriate care to the patient, or active (anything requiring current management) or inactive (prior problems that are resolved) problems. They are listed by priority according to the patient's current diagnosis.

The components of the POMR include:

- baseline data
  - ○ patient's health history, including medical, social, and emotional status
  - ○ initial assessment findings
  - ○ diagnostic test results
- problem list (formulated from baseline data)
- plan of care for each problem
- progress notes.

Focusing on each problem

The care plan in a POMR addresses each of the patient's problems, which are routinely updated in the plan and the progress notes.

Other medical record formats

Some facilities modify the source-oriented or problem-oriented method of documentation to suit their needs. If your facility does this, you're in a position to influence the type and style of documentation you use in medical records.

Designer documentation

For example, home health care nurses have created many specialized documentation forms or computer screens—including an initial assessment form, problem list, day-visit sheet, and discharge summary—to reflect the unique services and the essential quality of care they provide in order to meet their documentation needs while complying with state and federal laws and other regulations.

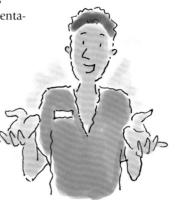

Whatever format you use, documentation should reflect the quality of nursing care you deliver.

A close look at a medical record

Although each health care facility has its own system for keeping medical records, most records (paper and electronic) contain the information described here:

• face sheet—contains the patient's name, birth date, social security number, address, marital status, closest relative or guardian, food and drug allergies, admitting diagnosis, attending practitioner, and insurance information

• conditions of admission form

• advance directives—living will or physician orders for life-sustaining treatment (POLST) which communicates end-of-life decisions

   – health care power of attorney form

• medical history and physical examination—completed by the practitioner; contains the initial medical examination and evaluation data

• practitioner's order sheet—a record of the practitioner's medical orders; may include orders by established protocol

• admission nursing assessment—contains patient data, including patient and family health history; medication reconciliation; physical assessment findings; and cultural, spiritual, psychosocial, and educational needs

• integrated assessment—assessment information documented by the multidisciplinary health care team

• problem or nursing diagnosis list—lists the patient's problems (used with problem-oriented medical records)

• nursing care plan—based on information gathered during patient assessment; specifies patient care needs and goals, planned interventions, and the patient's progress toward meeting goals and objectives

• education record—description of education provided, participants in education (e.g., patient or family), and level of understanding or need for further reinforcement

• vital signs—record of the patient's temperature, pulse, respiratory rate, blood pressure, and pulse oximetry

   – admission and daily weight (if required)

   – intake and output (if ordered)

• medication administration record—lists medications the patient is ordered and receives, including dosage, administration route, site, date, and time

• nursing assessment and care—details patient assessment as required by facility based on acuity, nursing interventions, and patient responses

• practitioner's progress notes—contains practitioners' observations, notes on the patient's progress, and treatment data (including consultants)

• diagnostic findings—contains diagnostic and laboratory data or point of care testing

• health care team records—includes information from the multidisciplinary team, such as the physical therapist, respiratory therapist, case manager, social worker, nutritionist, and other team members

• photographs—usually of wounds, such as a pressure injury

• discharge plan and summary—presents a brief account of the patient's time in the facility and plan of care after discharge.

Electronic health record

Electronic documentation of information is popular for completing medical records from admission through discharge. Called an "electronic health record" or EHR, this system of documentation has several benefits:

• It promotes standardization.

• Legibility problems that accompany handwritten entries are eliminated.

• Fewer errors may be made.

• It leads to decreased recording time and costs.

• Communication among team members is aided.

- It allows easier access to medical data for education, research, and performance improvement.

They even have good bedside manners

Information filed electronically may include nursing care plans, progress notes, medication records, records of vital signs, intake and output sheets, treatments provided, test results, and patient classifications. Some facilities even have bedside computers for quick data entry and access. One of the drawbacks of computerized documentation is the potential for unauthorized personnel to access confidential medical records. However, the electronic security provisions of the Health Insurance Portability and Accountability Act of 1996 (HIPAA) are meant to prevent this from occurring. These provisions prohibit clinicians from using facility computers for recreation, shopping, or other pursuits not related to patient care. Refraining from these activities will help safeguard computers from computer viruses that could allow unauthorized access to confidential information. (See *Super-successful electronic documentation.*)

For more information about computerized documentation, see chapter 4, Documentation systems.

That's a wrap!

Review of documentation basics

Roles of documentation
- Serves as a medium of communication for the health care team
- Can be used in health care evaluations
- Serves as legal evidence
- Can be used to aid research and education
- Helps facilities obtain accreditation and licensure
- Provides justification for reimbursement
- Is used to develop improvements in the quality of care
- Indicates compliance with your state's nurse practice act
- Establishes professional accountability

Types of medical records
- Source-oriented—has separate sections for each discipline's documentation, which keeps team members from getting the complete picture and breaks down communication
- Problem-oriented—is based on the patient's acute and chronic medical problems and contains baseline data from all departments

Electronic health record
- Promotes standardization
- Eliminates legibility problems
- Leads to decreased recording time and costs
- Aids team communication
- Allows easier access to medical data

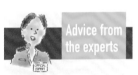

Advice from the experts

Super-successful electronic documentation

To be effective, an electronic documentation system must:
- record and send data to the appropriate department
- adapt easily to the health care facility's needs
- display highly selective information on command
- provide easy access and retrieval for all trained personnel.

Suggested references

American Nurses Association. "ANA's Principles for Nursing Documentation: Guidance for Registered Nurses," 2010. Available: http://www.nursingworld.org/principles.

Austin, S. "Stay out of court with proper documentation," *Nursing2011* 41(4):24-29, April 2011.

Centers for Medicare & Medicaid Services. "Design and Development of the Diagnosis Related Group (DRG)," 2016. Available: https://www.cms.gov/ICD10Manual/version34-fullcode-cms/fullcode_cms/Design_and_development_of_the_Diagnosis_Related_Group_(DRGs)_PBL-038.pdf.

Centers for Medicare & Medicaid Services. "Electronic Health Records," 2012. Available: https://www.cms.gov/Medicare/E-Health/EHealthRecords/index.html.

Chapter 2

The nursing process

Just the facts

In this chapter, you'll learn:

♦ guidelines for performing an assessment based on the nursing process

♦ methods for formulating a nursing diagnosis

♦ ways to write nursing care plans with expected outcomes and appropriate interventions

♦ evaluation and documentation of nursing interventions and outcomes.

A look at the nursing process

The nursing process is a problem-solving approach to nursing care. It's a systematic and rational method of providing care for a patient by utilizing critical thinking while assessing a patient, determining problems, devising a plan of care to address them, implementing the plan, and evaluating the effectiveness of the care provided.

The roots of the nursing process can be traced to World War II. By the 1960s, however, technology, medical advances, and a growing need for nurses began to change the nursing profession. It was at this time, as team health care came into wider practice and nurses were increasingly called on to define their specific roles, that the nursing process emerged.

Going through the steps

The nursing process consists of five distinct steps:

1. assessment
2. nursing diagnosis
3. planning care/outcomes
4. implementation
5. evaluation.

These five steps are dynamic and flexible, with some overlap. They work together to guide the nurse to identify and correct patient problems.

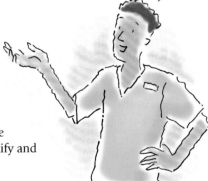

The nursing process is a five-step circular path from assessment to evaluation and then back to assessment.

Nursing Process

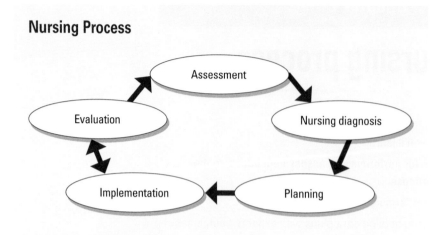

Assessment → Nursing diagnosis → Planning → Implementation → Evaluation → Assessment

Assessment

The first step in the nursing process—assessment—begins as soon as you come in contact with the patient. Assessment continues throughout the patient's hospitalization with every encounter and with any change in the patient's condition.

Getting the whole picture

Assessment is the collection of relevant information (data) from various sources (including the patient) and analyzing it to form a complete picture of your patient. As you collect this information, you need to document it accurately for two reasons:

- It guides you through the rest of the nursing process, helping you formulate nursing diagnoses, nursing interventions, and expected outcomes.
- It serves as a vital communication tool for other team members and as a baseline for evaluating a patient's progress.

The information that you gather at any point while caring for the patient may indicate that a broader or more detailed assessment, such as a nutritional assessment, is needed. (See *Assessing nutritional status*, page 15.)

Further assessment depends on the:
- patient's diagnosis
- care setting
- patient's consent to treatment
- care the patient is seeking
- patient's response to previous care.

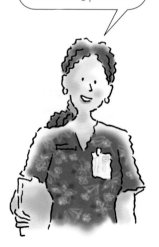

The assessment data that I collect helps establish the basis for the rest of the nursing process.

Assessing nutritional status

As part of the health history, the answers to some questions automatically call for another discipline to be consulted. An example is the nutrition history.

With the following questions, one "no" requires a nutritional consult:
* Do you have sufficient funds to buy food?
* Do you have access to a food market?
* Can you shop, cook, and feed yourself?

With the following questions, one "yes" requires a nutritional consult:
* Do you have an illness or condition that made you change the amount or kind of food you eat?
* Do you have dental or mouth problems that make it difficult for you to chew or swallow food?
* Do you need help getting to a food market?
* Have you lost or gained 10 lb within the past 6 months without trying?

First impressions

In your initial assessment, consider the patient's immediate and emerging needs, including not only physical needs but also psychological, spiritual, social, and educational concerns. Your first assessment of the patient helps you determine what care the patient needs and sets the stage for additional assessments. Remember that a patient's family, culture, and religion are important factors in the patient's response to illness and treatment.

Begin your assessment by collecting or reviewing the patient's health history and conducting a physical examination.

Health history

The health history is a patient interview to collect physical, psychological, cultural, spiritual, and psychosocial data. It's the main source of information about the patient's health status and guides the physical examination that follows.

The patient's health history is typically collected on admission to a facility and can help all the nurses caring for the patient focus holistically on the human response to illness.

The health history collected helps:
* identify problems
* plan health care

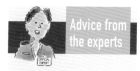

Advice from the experts

Review health history

If the health history is already completed before your first encounter with the patient, review it for any information that may assist with your assessment of the patient.

- assess the impact of illness on the patient and members of the family
- evaluate the patient's health education needs
- initiate discharge planning.

Getting started

Although nurses conduct health histories in different ways, all interviews must progress in a logical sequence and the nurse must document the patient's response in an organized way. Most facilities provide specific forms or computerized screens that help direct the interview and document the provided information.

Before conducting the health history, consider the patient's ability to participate. If the patient's sedated, confused, hostile, angry, short of breath, or experiencing pain, ask only the most essential questions. Then perform an in-depth interview when the patient is better able or willing to cooperate or ask family members to provide information, as appropriate.

Get off on the right foot by greeting the patient and introducing yourself and explaining your role. Also greet any family members present and make them feel welcome. Be sure to ask the patient if it is permissible to conduct the interview with others present. Shut the door to the room to create a quiet, private space to make the patient feel as comfortable and relaxed as possible. Maintain eye contact to reassure the patient that you're interested in the conversation. Take the time to sit down if able and plan ahead to minimize interruptions. (See *Health history lessons*, page 17.)

Making the most of your time

Finding time to conduct a thorough health history is sometimes hard. However, a few strategies can help you keep interview time to a minimum without sacrificing quality. (See *Health history in a hurry*, page 18.)

Sometimes, an interview isn't even necessary—you can simply ask the patient to complete a questionnaire about past and present health status. Then you can quickly and easily document the patient's health history by reviewing the information on the questionnaire and filing it in the patient's medical record.

This method is most successful for patients who are to undergo short or elective procedures. The questionnaire can be completed before the patient's admission, which can save time.

In some acute care settings, modified questionnaires are used to evaluate language or reading problems the patient may have. The nurse then reviews sections that are completed by the patient.

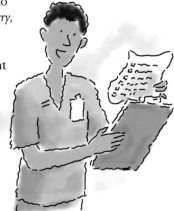

If a questionnaire saves time, I'm all for it!

Health history lessons

Conduct a health history with professionalism; when you show the patient that you're interested and empathetic, you elicit more accurate and complete answers.

Do

Here are some interviewing *do's*:

• *Ask open-ended questions.* Questions that require more than a yes-or-no answer encourage more individual expression. Ask, "Tell me more about your pain?" rather than "Are you still experiencing the pain in your leg?" Then move on to focused questions to gain more specific information.

• *Ask one question at a time.* Asking a question with multiple choices built in may cause confusion, such as "Do you have pain when walking, running, or climbing stairs?"

• *Avoid interrupting.* Allow the patient to answer questions fully to gain more information.

• *Restate information.* Summarize the patient's comments and then provide the opportunity for clarification.

Don't

Here are some interviewing *don'ts*:

• *Ask judgmental or threatening questions.* Saying "Why did you do that?" or "Explain your behavior" forces the patient to justify feelings or actions and might create alienation. The patient might even invent an appropriate answer just to satisfy you.

• *Ask persistent questions or probe.* Make one or two attempts to get information and then back off. Respect the patient's right to privacy.

• *Offer advice or false reassurance.* Giving advice implies that you know what's best for the patient. Instead, encourage the patient to participate in health care decisions. Saying "You'll be all right" devalues the patient's feelings, but saying "You seem worried" encourages candid conversation.

Physical examination

The assessment process also involves performing a physical examination. Use the following techniques to conduct the examination:

• inspection
• palpation
• percussion
• auscultation.

The objective data you gather during the physical examination may be used to confirm or rule out health problems that were suggested or suspected during the health history. You rely on these findings when you develop a care plan and when you provide patient teaching. For example, if the patient's blood pressure is high, you may need to provide teaching regarding a sodium-restricted diet and instruction on how to control hypertension.

It's in the details

How detailed should your examination be? That depends on the patient's condition, the clinical setting, and the policies and procedures

Health history in a hurry

When you're pressed for time, use the following tips to speed up health history documentation:

• Before the interview, fill in as much information as you can from admission forms, transfer summaries, and the medical history to avoid duplicating efforts. If information isn't clear, ask the patient for more details. For instance, you might say, "You told Dr. Brown that you sometimes feel like you can't catch your breath. Can you tell me more about when this happens?"

• Check your facility's policy on who may gather assessment data. Maybe you can have an unlicensed nursing assistant or technician collect routine information, such as allergies and past hospitalizations. Remember, however, that reviewing and verifying the information is your responsibility.

• Begin by asking about the patient's chief complaint. Then, even if the interview is interrupted, you'll still be able to begin developing a care plan.

• Use your facility's nursing assessment documentation form as a guide to organizing information. Ask your patient only pertinent questions from the form.

• Take only brief notes during the interview so you don't interrupt the flow of conversation. Write detailed notes as soon as possible after the interview. You can always go back to the patient if you need to clarify or verify information.

• Record your findings in concise, specific phrases or in specific fields detailed by computerized screens.

• Use only approved abbreviations, symbols, and acronyms. Review your facility's policy and The Joint Commission's "Do Not Use" abbreviation list. (See chapter 6, pages 120 to 154, for more information.)

established by your health care facility. The main components of the physical examination include:
• height
• weight
• vital signs
• pain
• review of the major body systems. (See *Rapid review of the physical assessment*, page 19.)

The Joint Commission standards

Under the standards of The Joint Commission, your initial assessment of the patient should consider:
• *physical factors*
• *psychological, social, and cultural factors*
• *nutritional and hydration status*
• *environmental factors*
• *self-care capabilities*

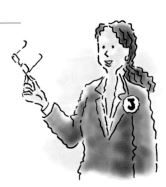

Rapid review of the physical assessment

During a physical examination, the major body systems are examined and evaluated. Pain also needs to be assessed as it applies to each system. Here's a typical body system review for an adult patient.

Respiratory system
Note the rate and rhythm of respirations and auscultate the lung fields. Watch for flaring or retractions as the patient breathes. Inspect the lips, mucous membranes, and nail beds. Also inspect the sputum, noting color, consistency, and other characteristics. Note pulse oximetry reading, if available.

Cardiovascular system
Note the patient's pulse and if it is high or low, weak, thready, or bounding. Also assess whether it is regular or irregular. Note the color and temperature of the extremities and assess the peripheral pulses. Check for edema and hair loss on the extremities. Inspect the neck veins and auscultate for heart sounds and regularity.

Neurologic system
Assess the patient's level of consciousness, noting orientation to time, place, and person and ability to follow commands. Also assess pupillary reactions. Check the extremities for movement and sensation.

Eyes, ears, nose, and throat
Assess the patient's ability to see objects with and without corrective lenses. Assess the patient's ability to hear spoken words clearly. Inspect the eyes and ears for

discharge and the nasal mucous membranes for dryness, irritation, and blood. Inspect the teeth, gums, tongue, and condition of the oral mucous membranes and palpate the lymph nodes in the neck.

Gastrointestinal system
Auscultate for bowel sounds in all quadrants. Note abdominal distention or ascites. Gently palpate the abdomen for tenderness. Note whether the abdomen is soft, hard, or distended.

Musculoskeletal system
Assess the range of motion of major joints. Look for swelling at the joints, contractures, muscle atrophy, or obvious deformity. Assess muscle strength of the trunk and extremities. Assess for pain with movement or palpation.

Genitourinary and reproductive systems
Note any bladder distention or incontinence. If indicated, inspect the genitalia for rashes, edema, injury, or deformity. (Inspection of the genitalia may be waived at the patient's request or if no dysfunction was reported during the interview.) Also examine the breasts, noting any abnormalities.

Integumentary system
Note the patient's skin color and temperature. Assess skin turgor and moisture or dryness. Note any petechiae, bruising, or discolorations. Assess breaks or abnormalities in the skin's integrity, such as abrasions, cuts, sores, lesions, scabs, plaques, scars, pressure injury, or rashes.

- *learning needs*
- *discharge planning needs*
- *input from the patient's family and friends when appropriate.*

Physical factors
Physical factors include the physical examination findings from your review of the patient's major body systems. Pain is usually the patient's main concern. Be sure to evaluate pain as part of the physical assessment.

Pain

The Joint Commission requires assessment and management of a patient's pain. Assess patients for pain during your initial assessment and in accordance to your hospital's policy. Choose an assessment method based on patient factors, including age and cognition. Reassess pain and document treatment and responses to treatment. Include the patient in identifying nonpharmacologic and pharmacologic treatment methods that may help manage the pain.

Factors affecting the patient

The patient's fears, anxieties, and other concerns about hospitalization may involve family, environmental, financial, psychological, and cultural factors.

Family matters

Find out what support systems the patient has by asking such questions as "How does being in the hospital affect your home situation?" A patient who's worried about family might be less able or willing to comply with treatment. Ask about child care concerns or if the patient is caring for parents or a sick spouse. The patient may put family matters above personal care, thereby complicating care. Identification of needs may prompt a social service consult to provide assistance that the patient did not know was available.

Abuse or neglect

Assess patients for signs of abuse or neglect. Know your role in reporting any suspicion internally and as required by law or regulation to an external agency.

Environmental factors

The patient's home environment affects care needs during hospitalization and after discharge. Factors to ask about may include:

- where the patient lives and the type of housing (house or apartment)
- whether the patient has adequate heat, ventilation, hot water, and bathroom facilities
- how many flights of stairs the patient needs to climb
- whether the layout of the home poses any hazards
- whether there are pets in the home
- whether the home is convenient to stores and practitioners' offices.

Is the patient well-equipped?

In addition, ask if the patient uses equipment that isn't available in the hospital when performing activities of daily living (ADLs) at home. Tailor your questions to the patient's condition.

Self-care capabilities

A patient's ability to perform ADLs affects compliance with therapy before and after discharge. Assess your patient's ability to eat, wash, dress, use the bathroom, turn in bed, get out of bed, and get around. Some facilities use an ADLs checklist to indicate whether a patient can perform these tasks independently or whether assistance is needed.

Risk for falls

Screen your patient for falls risk. Use an assessment tool if provided by your organization. Consider the patient's history, comorbidities, medications, and current functional and mental status. Using this information, implement interventions to reduce your patient's risk for falls.

Financial factors

The patient may have anxiety concerning finances while hospitalized. Investigate how the illness or hospitalization affects the patient's job. Being incapacitated for even a short period may cause hardship for the patient and family. The patient may also be concerned about the hospital bill, especially if the patient does not have health insurance coverage. Case management or social services may be able to assist with this issue, decreasing the patient's anxiety.

Psychological factors

Review the patient's history for any psychological problems. Does the patient have a history of depression? Being hospitalized may exacerbate a previous problem or create a new one. Be aware of the patient's response to the stress of being ill.

Cultural factors

A patient's culture may affect the way a patient responds to care. At the first patient encounter, establish the patient's language needs. Obtain the assistance of an interpreter, if needed. Establish the patient's culture and learn what practices or expectations the patient has in regard to care. The patient may respond differently when addressed, touched, and treated appropriately. Also, culture may play a role in the patient's diet and routines. Be sure to investigate the patient's cultural habits if you are not already knowledgeable. (See *Identifying your patient's cultural needs*, page 22.)

Learning needs

Deciding early what your patient needs to know about the diagnosis and treatment leads to effective patient teaching. During the initial assessment, evaluate your patient's knowledge of the disease process, self-care, diet, medications, lifestyle changes, treatment measures, and limitations caused by the disease or treatment. Also, assess your patient's learning preferences—for example, does your patient like

(Text continues on page 24.)

Identifying your patient's cultural needs

A transcultural assessment tool can help promote cultural sensitivity in any nursing setting. Consult your facility's policy on the use of such forms, or incorporate the information included in this sample form when developing your patient's care plan.

Date _5/1/17_   **Time** _1015_   **Pt name** _Claudette Valiente_   **Age** _34_ ☐ M ☑ F
Medical dx: _36 weeks pregnant, states "high sugar in my blood"_

Communication (language, voice quality, pronunciation, use of silence and nonverbals)

Subjective data
Can you speak English?   ☑ Yes   ☐ No _____
Can you read English?   ☑ Yes   ☐ No _with difficulty_
Are you able to read lips?   ☐ Yes   ☑ No _____
Native language? _Creole_
Do you speak or read any other language? _No_
How do you want to be addressed? ☐ Mr. ☐ Mrs. ☐ Ms. ☑ First name ☐ Nickname _____

Objective data
How would you characterize the nonverbal communication style? _very open_
Eye contact: ☐ Direct   ☑ Peripheral gaze or no eye contact preferred during interactions
Use of interpreter: ☐ Family   ☐ Friend   ☐ Professional   ☐ Other   ☑ None
Overall communication style: ☑ Verbally loud and expressive   ☐ Quiet, reserved   ☐ Use of silence
Meaning of common signs—O.K., got ya nose, index finger summons, V sign, thumbs up
Understands above signs except "got ya nose"
Determine any familial colloquialisms used by individuals or families that may impact on assessment, treatment, or other interventions. _None noted_

Social orientation (culture, race, ethnicity, family role function, work, leisure, church, and friends)

Subjective data
Country of birth? _Haiti_   Years in this country? _3_
(If an immigrant or a refugee, how long has the patient lived in this country? —You are not questioning citizen status.)
What setting did you grow up in? ☐ Urban   ☐ Suburban   ☑ Rural
What is your ethnic identity? _Haitian_
Who are the major support people? ☑ Family members   ☐ Friends   ☐ Other _____
Who are the dominant family members? _Husband, grandparents_
Who makes major decisions for the family? _A family meeting is held_
Occupation in native country? _None_   Present occupation? _None_
Education? _Finished 6th grade_
Is religion important to you? _Yes_
What is your religious affiliation? _Catholic_   Would you like a chaplain visit? ☐ Yes ☑ No
Any cultural/religious practices/restrictions? If yes, describe _Balancing "hot" and "cold," believes_
in some voodoo passed down from mother and grandmother

Objective data
Interaction with family/significant other — describe _Animated, physically close, frequent touch,_
eye contact with family members
Age and life cycle factors must be considered in interactions with individuals and families (for example, high value placed on the decision of elders, the role of the eldest man or woman in the family or roles and expectation of children within the family). _Elders highly respected, children expected to be obedient and_
respectful
Religious icons on person or in room? _Wearing cross_

Identifying your patient's cultural needs (continued)

Space (comfort in conversation, proximity to others, body movement, perception of space)

Subjective data
Do you have any plans for the future? _No, believes God will guide her_
What do you consider a proper greeting? _Kissing and touch with family_

Objective data
☑ Tactile relationships, affectionate & embracing
☐ Non-contact
Personal space _Very close with family, maintains 2-3 foot distance from RN_

Biological variations (skin color, body structure, genetic and enzymatic patterns, nutritional preferences and deficiencies)

Subjective data
What type of food do you prefer? _Rice, beans, plantains_
What type of food do you dislike? _Yogurt, cottage cheese_
What do you believe promotes health? _Good spiritual habits, balancing "hot" and "cold," and eating well_
Family history of disease? _Malaria, high blood pressure, "sugar"_

Objective data
Skin color _Deep brown_   Hair type _Coarse_

Environmental control (health practices, values, definitions of health and illness)

Subjective data
What do you think caused your problem? _"Ate wrong foods."_

Do you have an explanation for why it started when it did? _"No."_

What does your sickness do to you; how does it work? _"I don't think anything is wrong, but the doctor does."_
How severe is your sickness? How long do you expect it to last? _"It will go away soon."_

What problems has your sickness caused you? _"The doctor says my baby is big. But, a big baby is a strong baby."_
What fears do you have about your sickness? _"I have no fear. I will have a healthy baby."_

What kind of treatment do you think you should receive? _"Eating healthy."_

What are the most important results you hope to receive from this treatment? _"A healthy baby."_

What are the health and illness beliefs and practices of the family? _Uses home remedies such as herbs to treat sickness_
What are the most important things you do to keep healthy? _"Eat well."_

Any concerns about health and illness? _"No."_

What types of healing practices do you engage in (hot tea and lemon for cold, copper bracelet for arthritis, magnets)? _"Avoiding spices because they bother the baby, balancing hot and cold"_

(continued)

Identifying your patient's cultural needs (continued)

Environmental control *(continued)*

Objective data

Describe patient's appearance and surroundings <u>*Patient is clean and neatly groomed. Appears slightly overweight.*</u>

What diseases/disorders are endemic to the culture or country of origin? <u>*Intestinal problems, malnutrition, STDs, TB, sickle cell anemia, htn, cancer, AIDs*</u>

What are the customs and beliefs concerning major life events? <u>*Pregnant women are treated as special. Father of the baby doesn't participate in the birth experience; this is "women's business."*</u>

Time (use of measures, definitions, social and work time, time orientation — past, present, and future)

Subjective data

Preventative health measures? ☐ Yes ☑ No

Objective data

Time orientation ☐ Present ☑ Past

History of noncompliance, missed appointments <u>*Often misses appts or arrives late*</u>

to read educational pamphlets or watch videos? This will help you prepare and individualize your education accordingly.

No yes-or-no answers, please

One way to evaluate your patient's learning needs is to ask open-ended questions, such as "What do you know about the medicine you take?" The response will tell you whether the patient understands and complies with the medication regimen or whether more teaching is needed.

Learning obstacles

You should also assess factors that can hinder learning, which can result from the patient's:

- illness, injury, or physical disability
- health beliefs; trust or mistrust of health care professionals
- religious beliefs
- educational level; reading ability or health literacy
- cognitive disorder
- developmental disability
- sensory deficits such as hearing problems
- language barriers
- stress level
- age

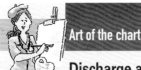

Art of the chart

Discharge assessment questions

The sample discharge assessment information below is important to know before the patient is discharged.

Discharge planning needs

Living arrangements (caregiver) *Going home with daughter, Sara Smith.*

Type of dwelling: Apartment ___ House ✓ Nursing home ___ Boarding home ___ Other _____

Physical barriers in home: No ___ Yes ✓ Explain: *12-step flight of stairs to bathroom and bedroom*

Access to follow-up medical care: Yes ✓ No ___ Explain: _____

Ability to carry out ADLs: Self-care ___ Partial assistance ✓ Total assistance ___

Needs help with: Bathing ✓ Eating ___ Ambulation ✓ Other *Medications*

Anticipated discharge destination: Home ✓ Rehab ___ Nursing home ___ Skilled nursing facility ___

- pain or discomfort
- motivation or readiness to learn
- cultural norms (may affect who the patient will take instruction from).

Discharge planning needs

Discharge planning should also start on admission (in some cases, even before admission), especially if the patient needs help after discharge. Find out where the patient will go after discharge. Is follow-up care accessible? Is there a caregiver who will be available to assist the patient? Are community resources, such as visiting nurse services and Meals on Wheels, offered where the patient lives? If not, you need time to help the patient make other arrangements. (See *Discharge assessment questions*.)

Prioritize, prioritize, prioritize

Because inpatient lengths of stay have become shorter and patient care has become increasingly complex, nurses must prioritize their assessment data. (See *Establishing priorities for patient assessment*, page 26.)

Input from family and friends

The Joint Commission requires that you obtain assessment information from the patient's family and friends when appropriate. When you interview someone other than the patient, be sure to document the nature of the relationship. If the interviewee isn't a family member, ask about and record the length of time the person has known the patient.

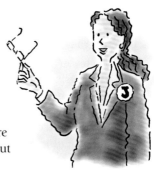

Establishing priorities for patient assessment

After completion of an initial assessment, The Joint Commission requires nurses to use the gathered information in prioritizing their care decisions. To systematically set priorities, follow these steps:
- Identify the patient's problems.
- Identify the patient's risk of injury.
- Identify the patient's need for help with self-care in the hospital and following discharge.
- Identify the educational needs of the patient and members of the family.

Nursing diagnosis

Your assessment findings form the basis for the next step in the nursing process: the nursing diagnosis. According to NANDA International (NANDA-I), a nursing diagnosis is a clinical judgment about individual, family, or community responses to actual or potential health problems or life processes. Nursing diagnoses are used in selecting nursing interventions to achieve outcomes for which the nurse is accountable.

Diagnosing a diagnosis

Each nursing diagnosis describes an actual or potential health problem that a nurse can legally manage. A diagnosis usually has three components:
1. the human response or problem—an actual or potential problem that can be affected by nursing care
2. related factors—factors that may precede, contribute to, or be associated with the human response
3. signs and symptoms—defining characteristics that lead to the diagnosis.

One patient, two types of treatment

When you become familiar with nursing diagnoses, you'll clearly see how nursing practice and medical practice differ. Although problems are identified in nursing and medicine, medical and nursing treatment approaches are very different.

The main difference is that practitioners are licensed to diagnose and treat illnesses, and nurses are licensed to diagnose and treat the patient's *response* to illness. Nurses can also diagnose the need for patient education, offer comfort and counsel to patients and families,

Maslow's pyramid

To formulate nursing diagnoses, you must know your patient's needs and values. Maslow's pyramid (shown below) illustrates those needs. Of course, physiologic needs—represented by the base of the pyramid in the diagram below—must be met first.

Self-actualization
Recognition and realization of one's potential, growth, health, and autonomy

Self-esteem
Sense of self-worth, self-respect, independence, dignity, privacy, self-reliance

Love and belonging
Affiliation, affection, intimacy, support, reassurance

Safety and security
Safety from physiologic and psychological threat, protection, continuity, stability, lack of danger

Physiologic needs
Oxygen, food, elimination, temperature control, sex, movement, rest, comfort

and care for patients until they're physically and emotionally ready to provide self-care.

Emergencies get top billing

Whenever you develop nursing diagnoses, you must prioritize them. Then begin your care plan with the problem with the highest priority. *High-priority* diagnoses involve emergency or immediate physical care needs. *Intermediate-priority* diagnoses involve nonemergency needs, and *low-priority* diagnoses involve peripheral needs or those related to enhanced functioning or wellness. Maslow's hierarchy of needs can help you set priorities in your care plan. (See *Maslow's pyramid*.)

Planning care/outcomes

The third step of the nursing process is planning care/outcomes. The nursing care plan is a written plan of action designed to help you deliver quality patient care. The care plan is based on problems identified during the patient's admission interview and can be modified as needed as the patient's hospital stay progresses. The plan consists of:
- nursing diagnoses
- expected outcomes
- nursing interventions.

Tips for top-notch care plans

Use either a traditional or standardized method for recording your care plan. A traditional care plan is written from scratch for each patient. A standardized care plan saves time because it's predetermined based on the patient's diagnosis. Additionally, a facility may utilize care plans that utilize research-based, standardized language established by NANDA International (NANDA-I) (nursing diagnoses), the Nursing Outcomes Classification (outcomes), and the Nursing Interventions Classification (interventions).

No matter which method you use, follow these tips to write a plan that's accurate and useful:
• Write in ink, sign your name, and include the date, if completing on paper or an established form.
• Use clear, concise language and not vague terms or generalities.
• Use standard abbreviations to avoid confusion.
• Review all your assessment data *before* selecting an approach for each problem. If you can't complete the initial assessment, immediately write *insufficient information* on your records.

• Write an expected outcome and a target date for each problem you identify.
• Set realistic initial outcomes.
• When writing nursing interventions, consider what to watch for and how often, what nursing measures to take and how to perform them, and what to teach the patient and family before discharge.
• Make each nursing intervention specific.
• Avoid duplicating or restating existing medical or nursing interventions.
• Make sure your interventions match the resources and capabilities of the staff.
• Record all of the patient's problems and concerns, so they won't be forgotten.
• Make sure your plan is implemented correctly.
• Evaluate the results of your plan and discontinue or complete nursing diagnoses that have been resolved. Select new approaches, if necessary, for problems that haven't been resolved. Add new diagnoses as needed.

The care plan becomes a permanent part of the patient's record and is used by all members of the nursing team. Remember, patients' problems and needs change, so review the care plan often and modify it if necessary.

Take three giant steps

Writing a care plan involves these three steps:
1. assigning priorities to the nursing diagnoses
2. selecting appropriate nursing interventions to accomplish expected outcomes
3. documenting the nursing diagnoses, expected outcomes, nursing interventions, and evaluations. (See *Tips for top-notch care plans.*)

Outcome identification

Part of the third step of the nursing process is outcome identification, which involves establishing individualized and measurable goals for your patient. The goal of your nursing care is to help your patient reach the highest functional level possible with minimal risk and problems. If the patient can't recover completely, your care should assist with coping physically and emotionally with impaired or declining health.

Keeping it real

Expected outcomes are goals the patient should reach as a result of planned nursing interventions. Sometimes, a nursing diagnosis requires more than one expected outcome.

You should identify realistic, measurable expected outcomes for each nursing diagnosis and set corresponding target dates to reach the goals.

An outcome can specify an improvement in the patient's ability to function—for example, an increase in the distance the patient is able to walk—or it can specify the correction of a problem such as a reduction of pain. In either case, each outcome calls for the maximum realistic improvement for a particular patient.

Four-part format

An outcome statement consists of four parts:
1. specific behavior that shows the patient has reached the established goal
2. criteria for measuring that behavior
3. conditions under which the behavior should occur
4. when the behavior should occur. (See *Components of an outcome statement*, page 30.)

Writing outcome statements

Save time when writing outcome statements by choosing your words carefully and being clear and concise. (See *Writing excellent outcome statements*, page 31.)

Here are some tips for writing efficient outcome statements:
- Avoid unnecessary words—For example, instead of writing *Pt will demonstrate correct wound-care technique by 5/1/18*, drop the first two words. It is understood that you're talking about the patient.
- Use accepted abbreviations—Refer to your facility's and The Joint Commission's official "Do Not Use" abbreviation lists as well as the Institute for Safe Medication Practices' "List of Error-Prone Abbreviations, Symbols, and Dose Designations." When using relative dates (describing the patient's stay in day-long intervals), use abbreviations such as *HD1* for hospital day 1 or *POD2* for postoperative day 2.

Components of an outcome statement

An outcome statement consists of four elements: behavior, measure, condition, and time.

    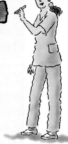

Behavior
A desired behavior for the patient; must be observable

Measure
Criteria for measuring the behavior; should specify how much, how long, how far, and so on

Condition
The conditions under which the behavior should occur

Time
When the behavior should occur

As indicated, the two outcome statements below have these four components.

Ambulate	one flight of stairs	unassisted	by 9/10/2017
Demonstrate	measuring radial pulse	before exercising	by 9/10/2017

- Make your statements specific—*Understand relaxation techniques* doesn't tell you much; how do you observe a patient's understanding? Instead, *Practice progressive muscle relaxation techniques unassisted for 15 minutes daily by 4/9/18* tells you exactly what to look for when assessing the patient's progress.
- Focus on the patient—Outcome statements should reflect the patient's behavior, not your intervention. *Medication brings chest pain relief* doesn't say anything about behavior. A correct statement would be *Express relief of chest pain within 1 hour of receiving medication.*
- Let the patient help you—A patient who helps formulate outcome statements is more motivated to achieve set goals. The patient's input, along with family member input, can help set more realistic goals.
- Consider medical orders—Don't write outcome statements that ignore or contradict medical orders. For example, before writing *Ambulate 10' unassisted twice a day by 6/9/18,* make sure that the medical orders don't call for more restricted activity, such as bed rest.
- Adapt the outcome to the circumstances—Consider the patient's coping ability, age, education, cultural influences, family support, living conditions, socioeconomic status, and anticipated length of stay. Also consider the health care setting. For example, *Ambulates outdoors with assistance for 20 minutes t.i.d. by 6/9/18* is probably unrealistic in a large city hospital.

Writing excellent outcome statements

The following tips will help you write clear, precise outcome statements:

• When writing expected outcomes in your care plan, always start with a specific action verb that focuses on your patient's behavior. By telling your reader how your patient should *look, walk, eat, drink, turn, cough, speak,* or *stand,* for example, you give a clear picture of how to evaluate progress.

• Avoid starting expected outcome statements with *allow, let, enable,* or similar verbs. Such words focus attention on your own and other health team members' behavior—not on the patient's.

• With many documentation formats, you won't need to include the phrase *The patient will . . .* with each expected outcome statement. You will, however, have to specify which person the goals refer to when family, friends, or others are directly concerned.

• Include realistic target dates for outcomes to help the patient and all health care team members track the patient's progress.

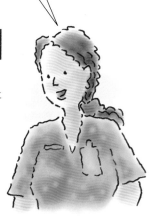

These guidelines will help you write great outcome statements.

Implementation

Now, you're ready to select interventions and implement them, the fourth step of the nursing process. Nursing interventions are actions that will help the patient reach the expected outcomes. Base these interventions on the second part of your nursing diagnosis, the related factors.

For example, with a nursing diagnosis of *Impaired physical mobility related to arthritic morning stiffness,* select interventions that reduce or eliminate the patient's stiffness, such as mild stretching exercises. Write at least one intervention for each outcome statement.

Divine intervention

How do you come up with interventions? There are several ways. First, consider interventions that you or your patient have successfully tried before. For example, if the patient is having trouble sleeping in the hospital and tells you that a glass of warm milk promotes sleep at home, this could work as an interventions of the expected outcome *Sleep through the night without medication by 11/9.*

You can also pick interventions from standardized care plans, ask other nurses about interventions they've used successfully, or check nursing journals for evidence-based interventions. If these methods don't work, try brainstorming with other nurses.

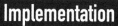

Writing interventions

To help you write interventions clearly and correctly, follow these guidelines:

- Clearly state the necessary action—Note how and when to perform the intervention and include special instructions. *Promote comfort* doesn't say what specific action to take, but *Administer ordered analgesic ½ hour before dressing change* says exactly what to do and when to do it.
- Make interventions fit the patient—Consider the patient's age, condition, developmental level, environment, ethnicity and culture, personal practices, and spiritual values. For instance, if the patient is a vegetarian, don't write an intervention that requires eating lean meat to gain extra protein for healing.
- Keep the patient's safety in mind—Consider the patient's physical and mental limitations. For instance, before teaching a patient how to administer medication, such as insulin injections, make sure that the patient can learn and follow the regimen and is physically capable of performing the task.
- Follow your facility's rules—For example, if your facility allows only nurses to administer medications, don't write an intervention calling for the patient to *Administer hemorrhoidal suppositories as needed.*
- Consider other health care activities—Adjust your interventions when other activities interfere with them. For example, you might want your patient to get plenty of rest on a day when there are several diagnostic tests scheduled.
- Use available resources—For example, if your patient needs to be educated regarding a specific cardiac problem, use your facility's education department, literature from the American Heart Association, educational media, and local support groups. Write your intervention to reflect the use of these resources.

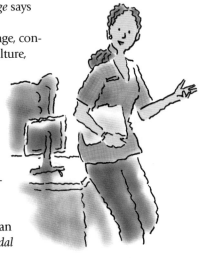

When writing interventions, clearly state the necessary action.

Documenting interventions

After you've performed an intervention, record the nature of the intervention, the time you performed it, and the patient's response. Also record other interventions that you performed based on the patient's response, the reasons you performed them, and the patient's response. Doing so makes your documentation *outcome-oriented*.

Tailor your style (and format) to policy

Where do you document interventions? That depends on your facility's policy. You can document them on graphic records, on a patient care flow sheet that integrates all nurses' notes for a 1-day period, on integrated or separate nurses' progress notes, on specialized documentation forms such as the medication administration record, or in electronic health records.

Your facility's policies also dictate the style and format of your documentation. You should record interventions when you give routine care, give emergency care, observe changes in the patient's condition, and administer medications.

Evaluation

The last step of the nursing process is evaluation. The current emphasis on evaluating your interventions has changed nursing documentation. Traditional documentation didn't always reflect the end results of nursing care, but today, your progress notes must include an evaluation of your patient's progress toward the expected outcomes you've established in the care plan.

Charting changes

The most commonly used charting method is expected outcomes and evaluation documentation. It focuses on the patient's response to nursing care and helps you provide high-quality, cost-effective care. It's replacing narrative charting and lengthy, handwritten care plans. (See *Effective evaluation statements.*)

A tough transition

The transition to outcome documentation has been difficult for some nurses. With outcome documentation, the nurse is expected to record nursing judgments, not just nursing interventions. Unfortunately, nurses have traditionally been trained not to make judgments. Today, nurses are being asked to gather and interpret data, refer and prioritize care, and document their findings.

The belief that hands-on care is more important than documentation is one reason nurses commonly focus more on nursing interventions than on documenting patient responses. However, worthwhile interventions lead to a desired outcome. Outcomes and evaluation documentation compels nurses to focus on patient responses. When you evaluate the results of your interventions, you help ensure that your plan is working or that adjustments are needed.

The value of evaluation

Evaluation of care gives you a chance to:
- determine if your original assessment findings still apply
- uncover complications or additional problems
- analyze patterns or trends in the patient's care and response to that care
- assess the patient's response to all aspects of provided care, including medications, changes in diet or activity, procedures, unusual incidents or problems, and teaching

Effective evaluation statements

The evaluation statements below clearly describe common outcomes. Note that they include specific details of the care provided and objective evidence of the patient's response to care.
- *Describes the signs and symptoms of hyperglycemia appropriately* (response to patient education)
- *States leg pain decreased from 9 to 6 (on a scale of 1 to 10) 30 minutes after receiving PCA morphine* (response to pain medication within 1 hour of administration)
- *Ambulates to chair with a steady gait, approximately 10', unassisted* (tolerance of change or increase in activity)
- *Dyspneic on room air even at rest; unable to tolerate oxygen removal* (tolerance of treatments)

- determine how closely care conforms to established standards
- measure how well you have cared for the patient
- assess the performance of other members of the health care team
- identify opportunities to improve the quality of your care.

Whenever within sight

Evaluation itself is an ongoing process that takes place whenever you see your patient. However, how often you're required to make evaluations depends on several factors, including where you work.

If you work in an acute care setting, your facility's policy may require you to review care plans every 24 hours. If you work in a long-term care facility, the required interval between evaluations may be as long as 30 days. In either case, you should evaluate and revise the care plan more often if warranted.

Evaluating expected outcomes

Evaluation includes gathering reassessment data, comparing findings with the outcome criteria, determining the extent of outcome achievement (whether the outcome was met, partially met, or not met), writing evaluation statements, and revising the care plan.

Not resolved? Revise . . .

Revision starts with determining whether the patient has achieved the outcomes. If outcomes haven't been fully met and you decide that the problem is resolved, the plan can be discontinued. If the problem persists, continue the plan with new target dates until the desired status is achieved. If outcomes are partially met or unmet, identify interfering factors, such as misinterpreted information, unrealistic patient outcomes, or a change in the patient's status, and revise the plan accordingly.

Revision may involve:

- clarifying or amending the database to reflect new information
- reexamining and correcting nursing diagnoses
- establishing outcome criteria that reflect new information and new or amended nursing strategies
- adding the revised nursing care plan to the original document
- recording the rationale for the revision in the nurses' progress notes.

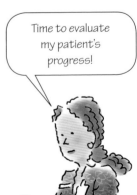

Time to evaluate my patient's progress!

Documenting evaluation

Evaluation statements should indicate whether expected outcomes were achieved and should list evidence supporting this conclusion. Base these statements on outcome criteria from the care plan and use action verbs, such as *demonstrate* or *ambulate*.

Get specific

Include the patient's response to specific treatments, such as medication administration or physical therapy, and describe the condition under which the response occurred or failed to occur. Document patient teaching and palliative or preventive care as well.

After evaluating the outcome, be sure to document it in the patient's medical record with clear statements that demonstrate progress, or lack of progress, toward meeting the expected outcomes.

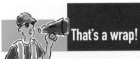

That's a wrap!

Nursing process review

Nursing process basics
- Problem-solving approach to nursing care
- Emerged in 1960s but its roots began in World War II (when the nursing profession began to change)
- Includes five steps: assessment, nursing diagnosis, planning care/outcomes, implementation, and evaluation

Assessment
- Guides the nursing process and communicates information to the health care team about the patient's condition
- Begins with a health history and physical examination
- Should follow The Joint Commission standards:
  - physical factors
  - psychological, social, and cultural factors
  - environmental factors
  - self-care capabilities
  - learning needs
  - discharge planning needs
  - input from the patient's family and friends when appropriate.

Nursing diagnosis
- Consists of the human response or problem, related factors, and signs and symptoms
- Must be formulated, prioritized, and then used to guide the care plan

Planning care/outcomes
- May be traditional or standardized
- Consists of nursing diagnoses, expected outcomes, and nursing interventions
- Used by all members of the health care team
- Involves assigning priorities, selecting nursing interventions, and documenting diagnoses, outcomes, interventions, and evaluations
- Should be modified if patient's condition changes
- Should include outcome identification with realistic, patient-focused, and measurable goals

Implementation
- Involves interventions, which help the patient reach expected outcomes and should be formulated with the patient's input, if possible
- Should be documented properly (interventions that clearly state the action, are individualized, address patient safety, adhere to facility policy, consider other health care activities, and use available resources)

Evaluation
- Consists of outcomes that include specific details about patient care and evidence of the patient's response to this care
- Includes gathering reassessment data, comparing findings, determining outcome achievement, writing evaluation statements, and revising the care plan, if necessary

Suggested references

American Nurses Association. "The Nursing Process," 2017. Available: http://www
     .nursingworld.org/EspeciallyForYou/What-is-Nursing/Tools-You-Need
     /Thenursingprocess.html.

Bickley, L.S. *Bates' Guide to Physical Examination and History Taking*, 12th ed. Philadelphia,
     PA: Lippincott Williams & Wilkins, 2016.

Herdman, T.H., and Kamitsuru, S., eds. *NANDA International, Inc. Nursing Diagnoses:
     Definitions & Classification 2015–2017*, 10th ed. Oxford, NY: Wiley-Blackwell, 2014.

Institute for Safe Medication Practices. "ISMP's List of Error-Prone Abbreviations,
     Symbols, and Dose Designations," 2015. Available: https://www.ismp.org
     /Tools/errorproneabbreviations.pdf.

NANDA International. "Knowledge-Based Terminologies Defining Nursing," 2017.
     Available: http://www.nanda.org/nanda-i-nic-noc.html.

The Joint Commission. *2016 CAMH Update 2: Comprehensive Accreditation Manual for
     Hospitals*. Oak Brook, IL: The Joint Commission Resources, 2016.

The Joint Commission. "Facts About the Official "Do Not Use" List of Abbreviations,"
     2017. Available: https://www.jointcommission.org/facts_about_do_not_use_list/

Chapter 3

Care plans

Just the facts

In this chapter, you'll learn:

◆ reasons for creating a care plan

◆ differences between traditional and standardized care plans

◆ functions and parts of a patient-teaching plan

◆ components of care pathways and their uses.

A look at the nursing care plan

For the health care team, the nursing care plan is a principal source of information about the patient's problems, needs, and goals. It contains interventions for achieving the goals established for the patient and is used to direct nursing care. It also includes suggestions for improving the patient's clinical problems and dealing with unexpected complications. Care plans incorporate critical thinking and prioritization in the delivery of holistic care for patients on a personal level. It details, organizes, and prioritizes the five Ws of care: who, what, why, when, and where, to help ensure continuity of care across the patient's caregivers and length of stay.

Because the care plan serves to organize and structure the team's care, without it, aspects of the patient care may be missed. Use of electronic health systems has made some aspects of documentation more comprehensive, but creation of an individualized care plan remains a pressing issue for the nurse caring for the patient.

Now a part of the permanent record

Until 1991, a care plan wasn't a required part of a patient's permanent record. It was used by the nursing staff, and in some facilities, it was discarded when a patient was discharged. *Now, The Joint Commission requires that the care plan be permanently integrated into the medical record by written or electronic means.*

However, The Joint Commission does not specify the format for documenting patient care plan, so many different methods are used. Most care plans follow the organizational steps of the nursing process. (See chapter 2, The nursing process.)

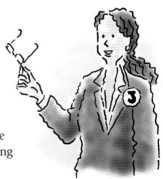

A word about words

Nurses lacked a standardized language to communicate their practice until the North American Nursing Diagnosis Association (NANDA) was introduced in 1973. Over time, more nursing languages have been developed, including (among others) the Nursing Minimum Data Set (NMDS), the Nursing Interventions Classification (NIC), and the Nursing Outcomes Classification (NOC) system. Critics state that nursing-specific language use does not always allow for flexibility and causes nurses to try to "fit" their patient's presentation into a known diagnosis. Use of a discipline-specific language can also lead to unnecessary confusion among the interdisciplinary team. Rather, many nursing professionals promote the use of more "common" language in writing care plans. As an example, many opt for the more common diagnosis of "pain" rather than "alteration in comfort, related to . . . ."

Whatever language is chosen for use by a facility or practitioner, it should be clear, complete, and concise and facilitates communication among the health care team and, ultimately, the patient.

Style of care plans

The care plan can be created in a *traditional* or *standardized* style. Either style should cover all identified patient problems and plan of care from admission to discharge.

Traditional care plans

Also called an *individually developed care plan*, the traditional care plan is written from scratch for each patient. However, the care plan may follow a standardized format, such as one that has columns for specific components, such as:

- nursing diagnoses
- expected goals or outcomes
- interventions
- evaluations.

There may be other columns for the date the care plan was initiated; target dates for expected outcomes; and the dates for review, revisions, and resolutions. Paper forms will also have a place for you to sign or initial whenever you make an entry or a revision. (See *It's a plan*, page 39.)

Electronic health records (EHRs) may automatically formulate a care plan based on documented assessment findings; however, it may need to be further individualized for your patient. The EHR will have some sort of electronic signature attached for identification of contributors to the care plan.

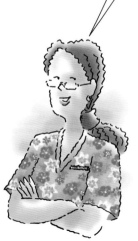

What's your style, traditional or standardized?

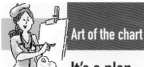

Art of the chart

It's a plan

Here's an example of a care plan. It shows how these care plans are typically organized. A care plan may be created from scratch for each patient or may be formulated electronically based on documented assessment findings.

Date	Nursing diagnosis	Expected outcomes	Interventions	Outcomes evaluation (initials and date)
7/15/2017	Ineffective breathing pattern R/T pain as evidenced by c/o pain with deep breaths or coughing	The patient will demonstrate respiratory rate within 5 of baseline and exhibit normal pulse oximetry readings and/or arterial blood gases values.	Assess and record respiratory status q4h. Assess for pain q4h and prn. Give pain medication as ordered and reassess pain within 30 minutes. Assist the patient to a comfortable position. Assist the patient in using incentive spirometry. Teach the patient how to splint chest while coughing. Perform chest physiotherapy to aid in mobilizing and removing secretions. Provide rest periods. Provide oxygen as ordered.	

> Nursing diagnoses, expected outcomes, interventions, and outcomes evaluations are key elements of traditional care plans.

Review dates

Date	Signature			Initials
7/16/2017	M. Hopper, RN			MH

Looking toward an outcome

Because shorter hospital stays are more common today, in most health care facilities, you're expected to write only short-term outcomes that the patient can reach by the time of discharge.

However, some facilities—especially long-term care facilities—also want you to identify long-term outcomes for the patient's maximum functioning level. These facilities commonly provide forms or computerized screens with separate spaces for short- and long-term outcomes.

Personal, visual, clear

The traditional method has several advantages:
- It provides a personalized plan for each patient.
- The format allows health care team members and the patient to easily visualize the plan.
- Columns for outcomes evaluations are clearly delineated.

Time isn't on its side

The main disadvantage of the traditional method is that it's time-consuming to write and read because it requires lengthy documentation. Additionally, if a paper form is used, legibility can become an issue when staff are rushed, use inappropriate abbreviations, or have poor handwriting.

Standardized care plans

Standardized care plans are more commonly used and were developed to eliminate the time constraints associated with traditional plans. Many patients with the same diagnoses share common problems. With this in mind, the standardized care plan is "prefilled" with common diagnoses, goals, and interventions to decrease documentation time. (See *Why stand on tradition? Use a standardized plan*, page 41.)

Some standardized plans are classified by medical diagnoses or diagnosis-related groups (DRGs), whereas others, by nursing diagnoses.

Insist on individuality

Even though it is standardized, this type of care plan also offers space for the nurse to explain how the plan is individualized for each patient by adding the following information:
- "related to" (R/T) and "evidenced by" statements for a nursing diagnosis that provide defining characteristics or related factors that support the diagnosis—If the form provides a root diagnosis, such as "Acute pain R/T _____," you might fill in *inflammation, as evidenced by grimacing and other expressions of pain.*
- time limits for the expected outcomes, such as— To a root statement of the goal *Perform postural drainage without assistance*, you might add *for 15 minutes immediately upon awakening in the morning, by 11/12/18.* Make sure that the outcomes are patient-centered and can be easily measured. (See *Penning precise patient outcomes*, page 42.)

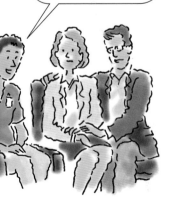

Each patient has unique needs.

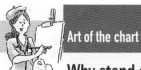

Art of the chart

Why stand on tradition? Use a standardized plan

The standardized care plan below is for a patient with a nursing diagnosis of *Impaired tissue integrity*. To customize it to your patient, complete the diagnosis—including signs and symptoms—and fill in the expected outcomes.

Date _7/15/2017_

Nursing diagnosis
Impaired tissue integrity _related to circulatory impairment_

> Standardized plans require a lot less writing.

Target date _7/17/2017_

Expected outcomes
Attains relief from immediate symptoms: _pain, ulcers, edema_
Voices intent to change modifiable risk factors: _will stop smoking immediately_
Maintains collateral circulation: _palpable peripheral pulses, extremities warm and pink with good capillary refill_
Voices intent to follow specific management routines after discharge: _foot care guidelines, exercise regimen as specified by physical therapy department_
Wound remains clean and demonstrates decreased drainage.

Date _7/15/2017_

Interventions
• Provide foot care. Administer and monitor treatments according to facility protocols.
• Encourage adherence to an exercise regimen as tolerated.
• Educate the patient about risk factors and prevention of injury. Refer the patient to a stop-smoking program.
• Maintain adequate hydration. Monitor I/O _q12h_
• Change dressing to foot ulcers daily and assess drainage for amount, color, and odor.
• Additional interventions: _inspect skin integrity q shift_

Date _____

Outcomes evaluation
Attained relief of immediate symptoms: _____
Voiced intent to change modifiable risk factors: _____
Maintained collateral circulation: _____
Voiced intent to follow specific management routines after discharge: _____

- frequency of interventions—To an intervention such as *Perform passive range-of-motion exercises,* you might add *twice per day: once in the morning and in the evening.*
- specific instructions for interventions—For the standard intervention *Elevate the patient's head,* you might specify *before sleep, on three pillows.*

Penning precise patient outcomes

Many nurses have difficulty writing specific outcomes, resulting in outcomes that are too generalized. Remember that your outcomes should clarify what the patient is expected to be able to accomplish and should be able to be measured in a specific time frame.

Compare the following two sets of patient outcomes.

Well-phrased outcome	Poorly phrased outcome
The patient with asthma will be able to maintain an effective breathing pattern as evidenced by relaxed breathing at a normal rate/depth and absence of dyspnea by the end of day 2 of hospitalization.	The patient with asthma will be able to report that breathing is better by discharge.
The patient with postop knee replacement will report that pain is at a "tolerable" pain level (3 to 4/10) by end of each shift.	The patient with postop knee replacement will have good pain control by discharge.

Computers make combos less cumbersome

When a patient has more than one diagnosis, standardized care plans must be combined, which can make records long, cumbersome, and sometimes confusing! However, if your facility uses computerized plans, you can extract only the parts you need from each plan and then combine them to make one manageable plan. Some computer programs provide a checklist of interventions from which you can select to build your own plan.

These advantages come standard

Standardized care plans offer many advantages because they:
- are less time-consuming
- are more understandable
- make compliance with a standard of care easier for all members of the health care team, regardless of level of nursing expertise
- guide the creation of the plan and allow you the freedom to adapt it to your patient.

Is it individualized?

This method has one main drawback: If you simply check off items on a list or fill in the blanks, you might not individualize the patient's care or document your findings adequately. This may create a void in providing information regarding nursing interventions provided to improve patient outcomes as well as a delinquency in following the standard of care required by regulatory agencies for accreditation. Special attention is needed to ensure that the care plan is complete and specific for each patient.

Interdisciplinary contributions to the care plans

When writing a clinical care plan, many nurses become confused about what interventions to include. For example, should they include the practitioner's orders, the occupational therapist's activities of daily living evaluations, the respiratory therapist's inhalation treatments, or the pharmacist's medications? Or, should they only include specific nursing interventions? When in doubt, include primary nursing interventions only, with a generalized statement related to evaluating the impact of the team's interventions. Also, follow your facility's guidelines.

Interdisciplinary care plans may help alleviate this issue. Interdisciplinary care plans are working documents that the entire team of health care professionals updates regularly. Each discipline provides interventions within their own specialty under each problem to show how the team is working together to achieve the desired outcome within a specified time frame. Members of the interdisciplinary team can also document when the patient has achieved the desired outcomes, providing feedback to the other members of the health care team as to the patient's condition related to their care. (See *Interdisciplinary care plan*, page 44.)

Patient-teaching plan

A patient-teaching plan is a nursing care plan that focuses on an essential component of care: patient and family education. It has many functions:
- It emphasizes the unique aspect of teaching/learning in improving the patient's health, compliance, and membership as part of the health care team.
- It pinpoints what the patient needs to learn and how it will be taught.
- It sets criteria for evaluating how well the patient learns.
- It helps all caregivers coordinate their teaching.
- It serves as legal proof that the patient received appropriate instruction and satisfies the requirements of regulatory agencies such as The Joint Commission.

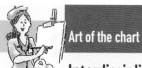

Art of the chart

Interdisciplinary care plan

The standardized care plan below is an interdisciplinary care plan that allows other members of the health care team to contribute to the care plan and evaluate outcomes for a patient with a nursing diagnosis of *Impaired tissue integrity*.

Date _7/15/2017_   **Nursing diagnosis**
Impaired tissue integrity _related to circulatory impairment_

> Standardized plans require a lot less writing.

Target date _7/17/2017_   **Expected outcomes**
Attains relief from immediate symptoms: _pain, ulcers, edema_
Voices intent to change modifiable risk factors: _will stop smoking immediately_
Maintains collateral circulation: _palpable peripheral pulses, extremities warm and pink with good capillary refill_
Voices intent to follow specific management routines after discharge: _foot care guidelines, exercise regimen as specified by physical therapy department_
(Wound care team) Wound remains clean and demonstrates decreased drainage.

Date _7/15/2017_   **Interventions**
• Provide foot care. Administer and monitor treatments according to facility protocols.
• Encourage adherence to an exercise regimen as tolerated.
• Educate the patient about risk factors and prevention of injury. Refer the patient to a stop-smoking program.
• Maintain adequate hydration. Monitor I/O _q12h_
• (Wound care team) Change dressing to foot ulcers daily and assess drainage for amount, color, and odor.
• Additional interventions: _inspect skin integrity q shift_

Date _____   **Outcomes evaluation**
Attained relief of immediate symptoms: _____
Voiced intent to change modifiable risk factors: _____
Maintained collateral circulation: _____
Voiced intent to follow specific management routines after discharge: _____

Pointers for the perfect plan

To make sure that your teaching plan is as effective as possible, consider carefully what the patient needs to learn, how you'll teach the patient, and how you'll measure the results. Work closely with the patient, members of the family or caregivers, and other health care team members to create realistic and attainable goals for your plan. Also provide for follow-up teaching during hospitalization and at home, if appropriate.

Be sure to keep your plan flexible. Allow for factors that may interfere with effective teaching, such as a patient's unreceptiveness because of a poor night's sleep or pain or your own daily time constraints.

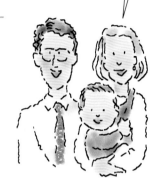

Make sure that you include us in your teaching plan.

Parts of the teaching plan

The patient-teaching plan is divided into six sections:
1. the patient's learning needs
2. expected learning outcomes
3. teaching content
4. teaching methods
5. teaching tools
6. evaluation of teaching effectiveness.

Learning needs

The first step in developing a teaching plan is to assess what the patient needs to learn. Sit with the patient to find out what is already known and what the patient expects to learn about the diagnosis and plan of care. Consider also what you, the practitioner, and other health care team members expect the patient to learn in order to be able to meet discharge and self-care needs. Adult learning theory tells us that people learn much better when they are both involved in identifying their needs and when they are invested in the outcomes—so prioritize the patient's desires first when teaching.

Learning outcomes

After you identify the patient's learning needs, you can establish expected learning outcomes, sometimes called *learning objectives*.

Like other patient care outcomes, expected learning objectives should focus on the patient and be easy to measure. Learning outcomes usually can be categorized into three different areas:
1. cognitive—relating to understanding
2. affective—dealing with attitudes and feelings
3. psychomotor—involving manual skills.

For example, for a patient who's learning to give self-injected medications, identifying an injection site is a *cognitive outcome*, coping with the need for injections is an *affective outcome*, and giving the injection is a *psychomotor outcome*. (See *Penning precise learning outcomes*, page 46.)

Which evaluation techniques are most valuable?

To develop precise, measurable outcomes, decide which evaluation techniques best reveal the patient's progress and write the outcome statement as it relates to this technique.

Penning precise learning outcomes

Learning behaviors fall into three categories: cognitive, psychomotor, and affective. Keeping these categories in mind will help you write clear, concise learning outcomes. Remember that your outcomes should clarify what you plan to teach, what behavior you expect to see, and what criteria you'll use for evaluating the patient's learning.

Compare the following two sets of learning outcomes.

Well-phrased learning outcomes	Poorly phrased learning outcomes
Cognitive domain	
The patient with heart failure will be able to teach back when and why to take each prescribed drug.	The patient with heart failure will be able to remember prescribed medications.
Affective domain	
The patient with heart failure will be able to talk about concerns and stresses related to the disease.	The patient with heart failure will be able to adjust successfully to the limitations of the disease.
Psychomotor domain	
The patient with heart failure will be able to demonstrate diaphragmatic pursed-lip breathing.	The patient with heart failure will be able to demonstrate easier breathing.

For cognitive learning, you might use questions and answer, or a technique called *teach-back*, where the patient explains what was understood. This can illuminate areas that need further clarification and can develop the patient's confidence when speaking about the diagnosis.

For psychomotor learning, the most effective evaluation method is a "return demonstration." This helps the patient to develop mastery of the skill and is an opportunity for the nurse to provide positive feedback and encouragement which often also positively impacts affective learning.

Measuring affective learning can be difficult because changes in attitude develop slowly. You may need to use several evaluation techniques. For example, you may want to encourage the patient to express all concerns and challenges to determine whether a patient has overcome feelings about anxiety about the diagnosis. You also can assess the patient's willingness to perform a skill or procedure and closely observe the patient's body language to identify signs of stress.

Content

Next, select what to teach the patient to help achieve the expected outcomes. Be sure to consult with the patient, members of the family, and other caregivers before deciding what to teach and how best to teach it. Even if the patient is learning self-care, it may be helpful to also teach a family member or caregiver how to provide physical and emotional support or how to help the patient remember what was taught. But before doing so, ask the patient's permission to involve others to avoid any infringements on privacy.

Start simple

After you have decided what to teach, organize your instruction to begin with the simplest concepts and work toward the more complex ones. Doing so is especially helpful when teaching a patient who has little education, a learning disability, or anxiety.

Methods

Now, select the appropriate teaching methods. Most of your teaching can probably be done one-on-one. Teaching one-on-one allows you to learn about your patient, build a relationship, and individualize your teaching to the patient's specific needs.

Taking different paths to learning

Many different teaching methods work well along with, or instead of, one-on-one teaching. For instance, try incorporating demonstration, practice, and return demonstration in your teaching plan. Role-playing can increase your patient's involvement in the plan, as can case studies, which require the patient to evaluate how someone else with the same disorder responds to different situations.

Other methods include self-monitoring, which requires the patient to evaluate the situation and determine which aspects of the environment or behavior need correction. You also can conduct group lectures and discussions if several patients require similar instruction, such as with breastfeeding or diabetes education.

Tools

Finally, decide what teaching tools will help enhance patient education. Before choosing your tools, involve the patient. Ask the patient what will work best to assist with learning. For instance, if your patient learns best by watching how something is done, use a videotape of a procedure or a closed-circuit television demonstration. (See *Tools for tuning up teaching*.)

If the patient prefers a hands-on approach, actual handling of the equipment may be the most effective way to learn. If the patient likes to work interactively, try an interactive, computerized patient-teaching program. If the patient learns best by reading, provide written materials. In some cases, using a variety of methods and tools is most effective.

Tracking down teaching tools

To get the tools you need, consult unit-based staff instructors, your facility's educational resource center, electronic teaching modules, and staff specialists. If you can't find what you need, call pharmaceutical

---

Tools for tuning up teaching

This list includes teaching materials and methods you can use to optimize your patient's learning.

Teaching materials

Teaching materials that may enhance learning include:
• brochures and pamphlets
• posters or charts
• DVDs and videotapes
• podcasts or YouTube videos
• computer programs
• models or images
• equipment being used for patient care (e.g., syringes, needles, and pumps).

Teaching methods

Teaching methods that may be effective include:
• one-on-one teaching
• role-playing
• return demonstration
• self-monitoring
• group class.

and medical supply companies in your community. Also, contact national associations and foundations such as the American Cancer Society. These organizations usually have many patient education materials written for the layperson. They also provide pamphlets and brochures in several languages.

Keep the patient's abilities and limitations in mind as you choose teaching tools. For example, before giving the patient written materials, such as brochures and pamphlets, evaluate reading ability and language or cultural barriers. Keep in mind that the average adult reads at only a sixth-grade level.

Break down language barriers

Assessment of language barriers between you and your patient should be identified on admission. For all teaching, use appropriate communication—including interpreter and translation services; bilingual aids, such as cards and pamphlets; and assistive listening devices—to overcome these barriers.

Evaluation

Evaluate the effectiveness of your teaching by using the technique you used for your expected learning outcomes. Document the patient's progress by documenting the patient's learning behaviors and indicating if the patient has met the expected learning outcomes.

Documenting the patient-teaching plan

The patient-teaching plan is a key part of the patient's care plan. By reading it, health care team members can see at a glance what the patient learned and what still needs to be taught or reinforced. The health care facility may also use it to determine the need for specialty programs or quality improvement projects.

Give it time . . . and thought

Constructing individual teaching plans requires time and thought. Ideally, health care team members collaborate to create these plans. However, because nurses typically spend more time with patients than other team members, they're usually responsible for individualizing standard teaching plans to meet each patient's needs.

Forms, forms, and more forms

There are several different types of forms or computer screens for documenting your patient-teaching plan. Many of these incorporate the nursing process as it applies to patient education. (See *Go with the flow sheet*, page 49.)

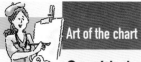

Art of the chart

Go with the flow sheet

Below is the first page of a patient-teaching flow sheet. Flow sheets like this one let you quickly and easily individualize your teaching plan to fit your patient's needs.

PATIENT-TEACHING FLOW SHEET

ASTHMA

Problems affecting learning

☐ None   ☐ Communication problem   ☐ Physical disability   ☐ Other _____

☑ Fatigue or pain   ☐ Cognitive or sensory impairment   ☐ Lack of motivation

> This form provides standard learning outcomes for patients with asthma.

LEARNING OUTCOMES	INITIAL TEACHING						REINFORCEMENT					
	Date	Time	Learner	Techniques and tools	Evaluation	Initials	Date	Time	Learner	Techniques and tools	Evaluation	Initials
Basic knowledge												
• Define asthma.	9/10/2017	1100	P	E,W	Dv	CB	9/11/2017	1100	P	E,W	S	CB
• List two symptoms of asthma.	9/10/2017	1100	P	E,W	Dv	CB	9/11/2017	1100	P	E,W	S	CB
Medication												
• State the action of theophylline and its effects on the body.	9/10/2017	1100	P	E,W	S	CB						
• Name the two inhalers used. Give their onsets, peaks, and durations.	9/10/2017	1100	P	E,W,V	Dv	CB						
• Demonstrate the ability to correctly use the inhalers.	9/10/2017	1100	P	E,W	S	CB						

KEY			
Learner	**Teaching techniques**	**Evaluation**	Signature: *Cindy Barton*
P = patient	D = demonstration	S = states understanding	Initials *CB*
S = spouse	E = explanation	D = demonstrates understanding	
M = mother	R = role playing	Dp = demonstrates understanding	
F = father		with physical coaching	
D1 = daughter 1 ____	**Teaching tools**	Dv = demonstrates understanding	
D2 = daughter 2 ____	F = filmstrip	with verbal coaching	
S1 = son 1 ____	P = physical model	T = passes written test	
S2 = son 2 ____	S = slide	N = no indication of learning	
O = other ____	V = videotape	NE = not evaluated	
	W = written material		

Just your type

Patient-teaching plans also come in two basic types that are similar to traditional and standardized care plans. The traditional type begins with the nursing diagnosis statement *Deficient knowledge* and an individualized *related to* statement—for example, *Deficient knowledge related to low-sodium diet*. It provides only the format and requires you to come up with the plan.

The standardized type allows you to check off or date steps as you complete them and add or delete information to individualize the plan. It's best suited for patients who need extensive teaching.

Some plans include space for documenting problems that could hinder learning (such as denial), for comments and evaluations, and for dates and signatures, or you may need to include this information in your progress notes. No matter which teaching plan you use, this information becomes a permanent part of the patient's medical record.

Care pathways

Care pathways go by many different names: *clinical pathways, critical paths, interdisciplinary plans, anticipated recovery plans, care maps, interdisciplinary action plans,* and *action plans*. Although most nurses think care pathways are a relatively new concept, they are based on an idea generated in the 1950s! The aim of a care pathway is to enhance the quality of care across the continuum by directing evidence-based patient outcomes, increasing patient satisfaction, and optimizing the work of the team.

A *care pathway* is a type of interdisciplinary care plan that describes assessment criteria, interventions, treatments, and outcomes for specific health-related conditions (usually based on a DRG, such as acute myocardial infarction) across a designated time line. Care paths are evidence-based and show the expected outcomes common to most patients in the spectrum of the disease. They incorporate something missing from standardized care plans, in that they include a space to identify, monitor, and evaluate variances from this norm—thereby inherently incorporating individualization.

Practical when predictable

Care pathways are most useful in specific types of patient care situations. They work well with high-volume cases (meaning, the facility cares for a lot of patients with this particular problem) and in situations that have relatively predictable outcomes. When used with the specific intended patient population, care pathways can encourage continuity of care, ensure appropriate use of resources, and reduce the cost and length of stay.

However, complex situations with unpredictable outcomes normally aren't managed with care pathways. Additionally, the structure of a care pathway and the categories it contains vary among facilities and often among departments within the same facility! (See *Take the care pathway*, pages 53 to 56.) This can be controversial and cumbersome especially when transferring a patient from one unit to the other. (See "Here's where it gets complicated . . . .")

Accomplished a goal? Check it off!

Care pathways cover the key care events that must occur before the patient's target discharge date. These events have boxes for check off with date/time/initial lines when completed to simplify documentation. The events may include:
- consultations
- diagnostic tests
- treatments
- medications
- procedures
- activities
- diet
- patient teaching
- discharge planning
- achievement of anticipated outcomes.

A collaborative effort

Members of the health care team involved in providing care should collaborate to develop each care pathway. The goals of the care pathway should include evidence-based practices or, if these are not available, benchmarked practices identified by other facilities that have been successful. Goals should include:
- achieving expected patient and family outcomes
- promoting professional collaborative practice and care
- ensuring continuity of care
- ensuring appropriate use of resources
- reducing the cost and length of stay
- establishing a framework for instituting and monitoring performance improvement.

Determining the path

Appropriate categories in any care path are determined based on the patient's medical diagnosis, list interventions, and care guidelines. The medical diagnosis also dictates expected length of stay, daily care guidelines, and expected outcomes.

Some facilities use nursing diagnoses as the basis for care pathways, but this use is controversial. Critics argue that this format interferes with communication and the coordination of care among non-nursing members of the health care team.

A bundle of benefits

Care pathways are overall a benefit to nurses. Here's why:

- They eliminate duplicate charting. You only need to write narrative notes when a standard on the pathway remains unmet or when the patient needs care that's different than what's written on the form. Most pathways provide a place to document care alterations. With less time needed for documentation, staff are freed up to spend more time in hands-on patient care.
- With standardized orders or protocols, the nurse has the freedom to advance the patient's activity level, diet, and treatment when the patient meets criteria without waiting for a practitioner's order.
- Communication improves between members of the health care team because everyone works and documents on the same plan. All members of the team work collaboratively to achieve the desired outcome.
- Quality of care improves because of shared accountability for patient outcomes. Analysis of variance data allows for periodic quality review and refinement of the care pathway.
- Patient teaching and discharge planning improve. When care pathways are adapted and given to patients, patients are less anxious and more cooperative because they know what to expect and what's expected of them. Some patients even recover and go home sooner than anticipated.
- Patients have increased satisfaction because they have a specific role in the pathway and are more involved in their care.
- Pathways help team members determine the best and most effective treatment methods.

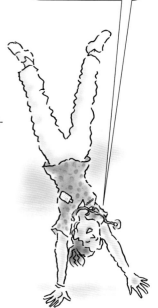

Care pathways improve my performance!

Here's where it gets complicated . . .

Even so, care pathways are less effective for patients who have several diagnoses or who have complications. Establishing a time line for these patients is more difficult. For example, treatment progress is usually predictable for a patient who has a cholecystectomy and is otherwise healthy. However, if a patient has diabetes and coronary artery disease, the treatment course is fairly unpredictable, and the care plan is likely to change, resulting in lengthy, fragmented documentation. Additionally, with a focus on minimal documentation, it is difficult to see the element of critical thinking in planning interventions and dealing with complications.

Choosing the right path

When a facility chooses pathways, they make sure that all disciplines have had a chance to provide input according to their specialty. Also, they plan to review pathways periodically to evaluate their usefulness

(Text continues on page 56.)

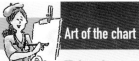

Art of the chart

Take the care pathway

At any point in a treatment course, a glance at the care pathway allows you to compare the patient's progress and your performance as a caregiver with standards. The standard care pathway below outlines care for a patient with a colon resection.

CARE PATHWAY: COLON RESECTION WITHOUT COLOSTOMY				
	Patient visit Date: _____	**Presurgery day 1** Date: _____	**Day 0 O.R. day** Date: _____	**Postoperative day 1** Date: _____
Assessments	History and physical with breast, rectal, and pelvic examinations Nursing assessment	Nursing admission assessment	Nursing admission assessment on TBA patients in holding area Postoperative review of systems assessment*	Review of systems assessment*
Consults	Social service consult Physical therapy consult	Notify referring practitioner of impending admission		CBC
Labs and diagnostics	Complete blood count (CBC) PT/PTT Electrocardiogram Chest X-ray (CXR) Chemistry profile CT scan ABD w/wo contrast CT scan pelvis Urinalysis Barium enema and flexible sigmoidoscopy or colonoscopy Biopsy report	Type and screen for patients with Hg level less than 10	Type and screen for patients in holding area with Hg level less than 10	

> The pathway designates a specific time frame for patient care activities.

(continued)

Take the care pathway *(continued)*

CARE PATHWAY: COLON RESECTION WITHOUT COLOSTOMY			
	Patient visit Date: _____	**Presurgery day 1** Date: _____	**Day 0 O.R. day** Date: _____	**Postoperative day 1** Date: _____
Interventions	Many or all of the above labs and diagnostics will have already been done. Check all results and fax to the surgeon's office.	Admit by 8 a.m. Check for bowel preparation orders Bowel preparation* Antiembolism stockings Incentive spirometry Ankle exercises* I.V. access* Routine VS* Pneumatic inflation boots	Shave and prepare in operating room NG tube maintenance* I/O VS per routine* Indwelling urinary catheter care Incentive spirometry* Ankle exercises* I.V. site care* HOB 30° Safety measures* Wound care* Mouth care*	NG tube maintenance* I/O* VS per routine* Indwelling urinary catheter care Incentive spirometry* Ankle exercises* I.V. site care* HOB 30°* Safety measures* Wound care* Mouth care* Antiembolism stockings
I.V.s		I.V. fluids, $D_5\frac{1}{2}$ NSS	I.V. fluids, D_5LR	I.V. fluids, D_5LR
Medication	Prescribe GoLYTELY or NuLYTELY 10a-2p Neomycin at 2p, 3p, and 10p Erythromycin at 2p, 3p, and 10p	GoLYTELY or NuLYTELY 10a-2p Erythromycin at 2p, 3p, and 10p Neomycin at 2p, 3p, and 10p	Preoperative ABX in holding area Postoperative ABX × 2 doses PCA (basal rate 0.5 mg) subcutaneous heparin	PCA (basal rate 0.5 mg) Sub Q heparin
Diet/GI	Clears presurgery day NPO after midnight	Clears presurgery day NPO after midnight	NPO/NG tube	
Activity			4 hours after surgery ambulate with abdominal binder* Discontinue pneumatic inflation boots once patient ambulates	Ambulate t.i.d. with abdominal binder* May shower Physical therapy b.i.d.
KEY: *= NSG **Activities** V = Variance N = No Var.	1. V Ⓝ 2. V N	1. V Ⓝ 2. V Ⓝ	1. V Ⓝ 2. V Ⓝ	1. V Ⓝ 2. V Ⓝ
Signatures:	1. *C. Molloy, RN* 2. _____	1. *M. Connel, RN* 2. *J. Smith, RN*	1. *L. Singer, RN* 2. *J. Smith, RN*	1. *L. Singer, RN* 2. *J. Smith, RN*

The pathway is organized into categories based on the patient's medical diagnosis.

The pathway lists tasks that the patient and caregivers must accomplish.

Take the care pathway *(continued)*

CARE PATHWAY: COLON RESECTION WITHOUT COLOSTOMY			
	Postoperative day 2 *Date:* _____	**Postoperative day 3** *Date:* _____	**Postoperative day 4** *Date:* _____	**Postoperative day 5** *Date:* _____
Assessments	Review of systems assessment*	Review of systems assessment*	Review of systems assessment	Review of systems assessment*
Consults		Dietary consult		Oncology consult if indicated (Dukes B2 or C or high risk lesion) (or to be done as outpatient)
Labs and diagnostics	Electrolyte 7 (EL-7) CXR	CBC EL-7	Pathology results on chart	CBC EL-7
Interventions	Discontinue nasogastric (NG) tube if possible* (per guidelines) Intake and output (I/O)* VS per routine* Discontinue indwelling urinary catheter Ambulating* Incentive spirometry* Ankle exercises* I.V. site care* Head of bed (HOB) 30°* Safety measures* Wound care* Mouth care* Antiembolism stockings	I/O* VS per routine* Incentive spirometry* Ankle exercises* I.V. site care* Safety measures* Wound care* Antiembolism stockings	I/O* VS per routine* Incentive spirometry* Ankle exercises* I.V. site care* Safety measures* Wound care* Antiembolism stockings	Consider staple removal Replace with adhesive strips Assess that patient has met discharge criteria* Discontinue saline lock
I.V.s	I.V. fluids D$_5$½ NSS+ MVI	I.V. convert to saline lock	Continue saline lock	Discontinue saline lock
Medication	PCA (0.5 mg basal rate)	Discontinue PCA P.O. analgesia Resume routine home meds	P.O. analgesia Preoperative meds	P.O. analgesia Preoperative meds
Diet/GI	Discontinue NG tube per guidelines: (Clamp tube at 8 a.m. if no N/V and residual <200 ml, discontinue tube at 12 noon)* (Check with doctor first)	Clears if+bm/flatus Advance to postoperative diet if tolerating clears (at least one tray of clears)	House	House

> The pathway also lists key events that must occur before the patient's discharge date.

(continued)

Take the care pathway *(continued)*

CARE PATHWAY: COLON RESECTION WITHOUT COLOSTOMY			
	Postoperative day 2 Date: _____	*Postoperative day 3* Date: _____	*Postoperative day 4* Date: _____	*Postoperative day 5* Date: _____
Activity	Ambulate q.i.d. with abdominal binder* May shower Physical therapy b.i.d.	Ambulate at least q.i.d. with abdominal binder* May shower Physical therapy b.i.d.	Ambulate at least q.i.d. with abdominal binder* May shower Physical therapy b.i.d.	
Teaching	Reinforce preoperative teaching* Patient and family education p.r.n.* Re: family screening	Reinforce preoperative teaching* Patient and family education p.r.n.* Re: family screening Begin discharge teaching	Reinforce preoperative teaching* Patient and family education p.r.n.* Discharge teaching re: reportable s/s, follow-up, and wound care*	Review all discharge instructions and Rx including:* follow-up appointments: with surgeon within 3 weeks with oncologist within 1 month if indicated
KEY: * = NSG Activities **V = Variance** **N = No Var.** **NSG care performed:**	1. 2. V V Ⓝ Ⓝ	1. 2. V V Ⓝ Ⓝ	1. 2. V V Ⓝ Ⓝ	1. 2. V V Ⓝ Ⓝ
Signatures:	1. *A. McCarthy, RN* 2. *R. Moyer, RN*	1. *A. McCarthy, RN* 2. *R. Moyer, RN*	1. *L. Singer, RN* 2. *J. Smith, RN*	1. *L. Singer, RN* 2. *J. Smith, RN*

and to ensure that the interventions are the most current evidence-based actions and that time lines are appropriate. Provide your suggestions for revisions as needed.

Priorities in the pathway

Just as you prioritize nursing diagnoses, you must prioritize collaborative problems in the care pathway. For example, if your patient needs whirlpool treatments by the physical therapist and nebulizer treatments from a respiratory therapist, you must coordinate these activities according to the patient's current status and needs. If every team member plans carefully and pays attention to the patient's response to treatments, you should be able to carry out your respective activities for the patient's benefit.

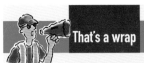

Care plans review

Criteria and language
- The Joint Commission requirements
- North American Nursing Diagnosis Association (NANDA), Nursing Minimum Data Set (NMDS), Nursing Interventions Classification (NIC), and Nursing Outcomes Classification (NOC)

Style of care plans
Traditional
- Advantages
  - Provides a personalized plan for each patient
  - Allows the health care team and patient to visualize the plan
  - Is clearly organized
- Disadvantage
  - Is time-consuming to read and write

Standardized
- Advantages
  - Uses preestablished information organized by diagnosis, which saves documentation time and facilitates adherence to facility standards
  - Requires less writing, which makes it easier to read
  - Is easier to duplicate
  - Guides care while allowing adaptability
- Disadvantage
  - May not be individualized properly if the nurse overlooks this important step

Patient-teaching plan
- Can be traditional or standardized

Functions
- To pinpoint what the patient needs to learn and how the patient likes to be taught
- To establish criteria for patient-learning evaluation
- To help caregivers coordinate teaching
- To prove that the patient received appropriate instruction

Parts of the teaching plan
- Learning needs
- Expected learning outcomes
- Content
- Methods
- Tools
- Evaluation

Care pathway
Basics
- Includes a predetermined checklist of tasks you and your patient must accomplish
- Provides daily care guidelines and expected outcomes
- Dictates the length of stay

Goals
- To achieve expected patient and family outcomes
- To promote professional collaborative practice and care
- To ensure continuity of care
- To ensure appropriate use of resources
- To reduce the cost and length of stay
- To establish a framework for instituting and monitoring continuous quality improvement
- To determine, over time, the most effective treatment

Advantages
- Eliminates duplicate charting
- Gives nurses more freedom in making care decisions
- Improves communication between members of the health care team
- Improves quality of care
- Improves patient teaching and discharge planning

Disadvantage
- Is less effective for patients with multiple diagnoses and those who experience complications

Suggested references

Beach, J., and Oates, J. "Maintaining Best Practice in Record-Keeping and Documentation," *Nursing Standard* 28(36):45-50, May 2014.

Keenan, G.M., et al. "Documentation and the Nurse Care Planning Process," 2008. Available: https://www.ncbi.nlm.nih.gov/books/NBK2674/.

Mannheim, J.K. "Choosing Effective Patient Education Materials," 2017. Available: https://medlineplus.gov/ency/patientinstructions/000455.htm.

RN Central. "What Is a Nursing Care Plan and Why Is It Needed?" 2017. Available: http://www.rncentral.com/nursing-library/careplans/.

Schrijvers, G., et al. "The Care Pathway Concept: Concepts and Theories: An Introduction," 2012. Available: https://www.ijic.org/articles/abstract/10.5334/ijic.812/.

Chapter 4

Documentation systems

Just the facts

In this chapter, you'll learn:

♦ different types of documentation systems and how to use them

♦ advantages and disadvantages of each type of system

♦ criteria to consider when choosing a documentation system.

A look at documentation systems

Different health care facilities set their own requirements for documentation and evaluation, but all must comply with legal, accreditation, and professional standards. A nursing department also may select its own documentation system as long as it adheres to those standards.

To write or not to write?

Depending on your facility's policy, you may use one or more documentation systems to record your nursing assessments, interventions, and evaluations of the patient's response. Although there are incentive programs for utilizing an electronic system of documentation, some facilities still use a traditional pen and paper documentation system. Others choose a combination of systems. There are pros and cons to each type of system.

Each system includes specific policies and procedures for documentation, so make sure you understand the documentation requirements for the system your facility uses. Understanding and adhering to these requirements will help you to document care systematically and accurately. (See *Comparing documentation systems*, page 60.)

Narrative documentation

Narrative documentation is a chronologic account of the patient's assessment findings and status, nursing interventions performed and the patient's response to those interventions. Today, few facilities rely on the narrative documentation system alone. Instead, they combine it with other systems, such as a narrative component and flow sheet system or a narrative component of the electronic health record (EHR).

Comparing documentation systems

The table below compares elements of the different documentation systems used today, with some being more popular than others. Note that the second column provides information on which systems work best in which settings.

System	Useful settings	Parts of record	Assessment	Care plan	Outcomes and evaluations	Progress notes format
Narrative	• Acute care • Long-term care • Home care • Ambulatory care	• Progress notes • Flow sheets to supplement care plan	• Initial: history and admission form • Ongoing: progress notes	• Care plan	• Progress notes • Discharge summaries	• Narration at time of entry
Problem-oriented medical record (POMR)	• Acute care • Long-term care • Home care • Rehabilitation • Mental health facilities	• Database • Problem list • Care plan • Progress notes • Discharge summary	• Initial: database and care plan • Ongoing: progress notes	• Database • Nursing care plan based on problem list	• Progress notes (section E of SOAPIE and SOAPIER)	• SOAP, SOAPIE, SOAPIER
Problem-intervention-evaluation (PIE)	• Acute care	• Assessment flow sheets • Progress notes • Problem list	• Initial: assessment form • Ongoing: assessment form every shift	• None; included in progress notes (section P)	• Progress notes (section E)	• Problem • Intervention • Evaluation
FOCUS (F-DAR)	• Acute care • Long-term care	• Progress notes • Flow sheets • Checklists	• Initial: patient history and admission assessment • Ongoing: assessment form	• Nursing care plan based on problems or nursing diagnoses	• Progress notes (section R)	• Data • Action • Response
Charting by exception (CBE)	• Acute care • Long-term care	• Care plan • Flow sheets, including patient-teaching records and patient discharge notes • Graphic record • Progress notes	• Initial: database assessment sheet • Ongoing: nursing and medical order flow sheets	• Nursing care plan based on nursing diagnoses	• Progress notes (section E)	• SOAPIE or SOAPIER
Electronic health record	• Acute care • Long-term care • Home care • Ambulatory care	• Progress notes • Flow sheets • Nursing care plan • Database • Teaching plan	• Initial: baseline assessment • Ongoing: progress notes	• Database • Care plan	• Outcome-based care plan	• Evaluative statements • Expected outcomes • Learning outcomes

Using narrative documentation

In the narrative system, the nurse usually records data as a progress note, with a flow sheet supplementing the narrative note. Knowing when and what to document and how to organize the data are the key elements of effective narrative documentation in the progress notes. (See *The full story on narrative documentation*.)

Documentation mania!

If you find yourself writing repetitious, meaningless notes, you may be documenting too often. If so, double-check your facility's policy. You may be following a time-consuming, unwritten standard initiated by staff members, not by your facility. To guard against this, review the policy at least every 6 months.

The Joint Commission requires all health care facilities to establish policies on the frequency of patient reassessment. So assess your patient at least as often as required by your facility's policy and then document your findings.

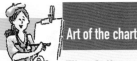

Art of the chart

The full story on narrative documentation

This progress note is one example of narrative documentation.

Date	Time	Notes
5/26/2017	1530	Pt lethargic but awakens easily; oriented x 3. Incision site in front of
		Ⓛ ear extending down and around ear and into neck – approximately 6"
		in length – dressing. Jackson Pratt drain in Ⓛ neck below ear with 20 ml
		bloody drainage measured. Drain and sutured in place and anchored to
		Ⓛ anterior chest wall with tape. Pt denies pain. c/o nausea, vomited 100 ml
		of clear fluid. Pt encouraged to deep-breathe and cough qh and turn
		frequently in bed. Antiembolism stockings applied to both lower extremities.
		Explanations given re: these preventive measures. Pt verbalized
		understanding. ———————————————————— Bridget Smith, RN
5/26/2017	1540	Pt continues to feel nauseated. Reglan 10 mg I.V. given ——— Bridget Smith, RN
5/26/2017	1600	Pt states she is no longer nauseated. No further vomiting. Continues to
		deny pain. Pt demonstrated taking deep breaths and coughing effectively.
		———————————————————— Bridget Smith, RN

Be sure to record the date and time of each entry.

Entries should be in chronologic order.

Remember to sign each entry.

Observe and take note

In addition to documenting assessments according to facility policy, be sure to write a specific and descriptive narrative in the progress notes whenever you observe:

- a change in the patient's condition, such as progression, regression, or new problems—for example, write *Patient can ambulate with a walker for 3 minutes before feeling tired*
- a patient's response to a treatment or medication—for example, write *Patient states that pain level decreased from a 7 out of 10 to 2 out of 10 in the pain scale (with 10 being the worst) pain*
- concerns regarding psychosocial issues, such as *Patient refused to speak to family members when visiting*
- a patient's or family member's response to teaching—for example, write *The patient was able to demonstrate walking with crutches using the proper technique.*

Be sure to document the date and time with each note, along with a signature, in order to confirm chronology of events.

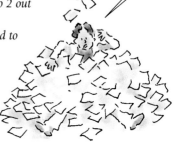

This is beginning to look all too familiar, not to mention meaningless. Am I documenting too much?

One thought leads to another

Before you write anything, organize your thoughts so your documentation flows smoothly. If you have trouble deciding what to write, refer to the patient's care plan to review:

- unresolved problems
- prescribed interventions
- expected outcomes.

Then write down your observations of the patient's progress in these areas. (See *Put your thoughts in order*, page 63.)

A narrative with a happy story

Narrative documentation has a lot going for it. After all, this documentation format:

- is the most flexible of all the documentation systems and is suitable in any clinical setting
- strongly conveys your nursing interventions and your patients' responses
- is ideal for presenting information that's collected over a long period
- combines well with other documentation devices, such as flow sheets, which cuts down on documentation time
- uses narration, the most common form of writing, so training new staff members can usually be done quickly
- places its narrative notes in chronologic order, so other team members can review the patient's progress daily.

Advice from the experts

Put your thoughts in order

If you have trouble organizing your thoughts, use this sequence of questions to order your entry:

* How did I first become aware of the problem?
* What has the patient said about the problem that's significant?
* What have I observed that's related to the problem?
* What's my plan for dealing with the problem?
* What steps have I taken to intervene?
* How has the patient responded to my interventions or medical regimen?

A paragraph for each problem

To make your notes as coherent as possible, discuss each of the patient's problems in a separate paragraph; don't lump them together. Alternatively, use a head-to-toe approach to organize your information.

Practitioner's orders

Be sure to notify the practitioner of significant changes that you observe. Then document this communication, the practitioner's responses, and any new orders to be implemented.

The narrative takes a turn for the worse . . .

On the other hand, narrative documentation has the following disadvantages:

* It is very time consuming to complete as well as to follow. Time spent on documentation means time away from caring for the patient.
* You have to read the entire record to find the patient outcome. Even then, you may have trouble determining the outcome of a problem because the same information may not be consistently documented.
* For the same reason, you may have trouble tracking problems and identifying trends in the patient's progress.
* Narrative documentation offers no inherent guide to what's important to document, so nurses commonly document everything, resulting in a lengthy, repetitive record.
* Narrative documentation doesn't always reflect the nursing process.
* Narratives may contain vague or inaccurate language, such as *appears to be bleeding* or *small amount.*
* Legibility may be a problem, resulting in problems associated with legalities or accreditation.

You may be able to avoid some disadvantages of narrative documentation by organizing the information you record. (See *AIR: A fresh narrative format*, page 64.)

AIR: A fresh narrative format

A documentation format called AIR may help you to organize and simplify your narrative documentation.

AIR is an acronym for:
- **A**ssessment
- **I**ntervention
- **R**esponse.

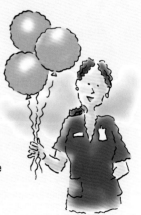

The AIR format synthesizes major nursing events and avoids repetition of information found elsewhere in the medical record. Combined with nursing flow sheets and the nursing care plan, the AIR format can be used to document the care you provide clearly and concisely.

Here's how AIR is used to document nursing care.

Assessment

Summarize your physical assessment findings. Begin by specifying each issue that you address, such as nursing diagnosis, admission note, and discharge planning. Rather than simply describing the patient's current condition, document trends and record your impression of the problem.

Intervention

Summarize your actions and those of other caregivers in response to the assessment data. The summary may include a condensed nursing care plan or plans for additional patient monitoring.

Response

Summarize the outcome or the patient's response to nursing interventions. Because a response may not be evident for hours or even days, this documentation may not immediately follow the entries. In fact, it may be recorded by another nurse, which is why titling each of your assessments and interventions is so important.

Problem–oriented medical record

The problem-oriented medical record (POMR) (also known as POR—problem-oriented record) focuses on specific patient problems and aids communication among team members. It was originally developed by practitioners and later adapted by nurses. The POMR is most effective in acute care and long-term care settings.

A multidiscipline approach

With this documentation system, you describe each problem in multidisciplinary patient progress notes (not on progress notes with only nursing information).

Four-part format

The POMR is divided into four parts:
1. database
2. problem list
3. plan of care
4. progress notes.

A four-star knowledge

With POMR documentation, you record your interventions and evaluations in the progress notes. However, to really understand POMR, review all four parts.

Database

Usually completed by a nurse, the database, or *initial assessment*, is the foundation for the patient's care plan. A collection of subjective and objective information about the patient, the database includes the reason for hospitalization, medical history, allergies, medication regimen, physical and psychosocial findings, self-care abilities, educational needs, and other discharge planning concerns. The database is the basis for a problem list.

Problem list

After analyzing the database, various caregivers list the patient's current problems in chronologic order according to the date when each is identified—not in the order of acuteness or priority. This list provides an overview of the patient's health status.

Dividing the diagnoses

Originally, POMR called for one interdisciplinary problem list. Although this may still be done, nurses and practitioners usually keep separate lists with problems stated as either nursing diagnoses or medical diagnoses.

It's as easy as 1, 2, 3, 4, 5 . . .

As you list the patient's problems, number them so they correspond to the problems in the rest of the POMR. Have every entry on the patient's plan of care and progress note correspond to a number. File the numbered problem list at the front of the patient's chart. Keep the list current by adding new numbers as new problems arise. When writing notes, be sure to identify the problem you're discussing by the appropriate number.

When you have resolved a problem, draw a line through it or show that it's inactive by retiring the problem number. Don't use the number again for the same patient.

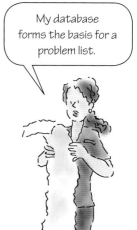

My *database* forms the basis for a *problem list*.

Plan of care

After constructing the problem list, write a plan of care for each problem. This plan includes:
- expected outcomes
- plans for further data collection, if needed
- patient care
- teaching plans.

Plan on patient participation

Involve the patient as much as possible in goal setting as you construct the plan of care. Doing so fosters the patient's compliance and is essential to the effectiveness of your interventions.

I want you to be involved in setting your goals in the initial plan.

Progress notes

One of the most prominent features of the POMR is the structured way that narrative progress notes are written by all team members using the SOAP, SOAPIE, or SOAPIER format. (See *SOAP, SOAPIE, SOAPIER documentation*, page 67.)

Usually, you must write a complete note in one of these formats every 24 hours whenever a problem is unresolved or the patient's condition changes.

A clean SOAP or SOAPIE component

You don't need to write an entry for each SOAP or SOAPIE component every time you document. If you have nothing to record for a component, either omit the letter from the note or leave a blank space after it, depending on your facility's policy. (See *Problem-oriented progress notes*, page 68.)

Sum it up

Prior to the patient's discharge, write a summary in the progress notes of each problem on the list and note whether it was resolved. This is the place in your SOAP or SOAPIE note to discuss discharge instructions provided, education provided and the patient and family understanding of the teaching, and if postdischarge arrangements are in place regarding home health care or follow-up appointments.

POMR pros . . .

The POMR documentation system has several advantages:
- Information about each problem is organized into specific categories that all caregivers can understand. This organization eases data retrieval and communication between disciplines.
- Continuity of care is shown by combining the care plan and progress notes into a complete record of care that's planned and care that's delivered. The caregiver addresses each problem or nursing diagnosis in the nurses' notes.

SOAP, SOAPIE, SOAPIER documentation

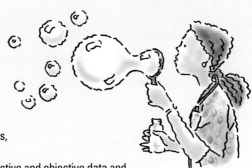

To use the SOAP format in problem-oriented medical record documentation, document the following information for each problem:
- **S**ubjective data: information the patient or family members tell you, such as the chief complaint and other impressions
- **O**bjective data: factual, measurable data you gather during assessment, such as observed signs and symptoms, vital signs, and laboratory test values
- **A**ssessment data: conclusions based on the collected subjective and objective data and formulated as patient problems or nursing diagnoses. This dynamic and ongoing process changes as more or different subjective and objective information becomes known.
- **P**lan: your strategy for relieving the patient's problem. This plan should include both immediate or short-term actions and long-term measures.

It's getting SOAPIE

Some facilities use the SOAPIE format, adding the following to SOAP:
- **I**ntervention: measures you take to achieve an expected outcome. As the patient's health status changes, you may need to modify your interventions. Be sure to document the patient's understanding and acceptance of the initial plan in this section of your notes.
- **E**valuation: an analysis of the effectiveness of your interventions

It's even SOAPIER

The SOAPIER format adds a revision section for the documentation of alternative interventions. If your patient's outcomes fall short of expectations, use the evaluation process called for in SOAPIE as a basis for developing revised interventions and then document these changes:
- **R**evision: Document any changes from the original care plan in this section. Interventions, outcomes, or target dates may need to be adjusted to reach a previous goal.

- It encourages nurses to document the nursing process, document more consistently, and document only essential data.
- It can be used effectively with standardized care plans, is an integrated medical record, and encourages collaboration of care among the health care team.

... and cons

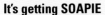

The POMR system also has some disadvantages, including the following:
- The emphasis on the chronology of problems, rather than their priority, may cause caregivers to disagree about which problems to list.
- Trends may be hard to analyze if information is buried in the daily narrative.

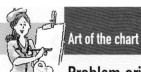

Art of the chart

No Problem!

Problem-oriented progress notes

The chart below is an example of progress notes as they appear in a problem-oriented medical record.

Date	Time	Notes
2/7/2017	0745	#1 Acute pain
		S: Pt states, "I am having severe back pain again and I'm nauseated."
		O: Pt states pain is #9 on 0-to-10 scale; skin is warm, pale, moist. Pt is restless, pacing in room, holding Ⓡ flank area with his hand.
		A: Pt in severe pain, needs medication for relief.
		P: Check orders for analgesia; check for any allergies; take VS; if within normal limits, give analgesia as ordered. Recheck pt in 30 minutes for response. Monitor pt for adverse reactions to drug. ———— Ann Davis, RN
2/7/2017	0805	#1 Acute pain
		S: Pt states, "The pain is less and I'm not nauseated."
		O: Pt states his pain is now a #2 on 0-to-10 scale. Skin warm and dry; color normal. Pt sitting on bed, watching the news.
		A: Pt has decreased pain.
		P: Continue to monitor for pain.
		I: BP 158/84, P 104, RR 24 – morphine 4 mg I.V.
		E: Medication was effective. ———— Ann Davis, RN
2/7/2017	1230	#2 Anxiety
		S: Pt states, "I am worried about the surgery and being out of work."
		O: Pt wringing his hands, eyes downcast.
		A: Pt is anxious regarding upcoming surgery and its impact on his job.
		P: Encourage verbalization of feelings and concerns. Offer emotional support. Involve family to discuss his concerns if agreeable to pt. ———— Ann Davis, RN
2/7/2017	1230	#3 Deficient knowledge
		S: Pt states, "I never had surgery before."
		O: Pt is unsure about what to expect from surgery.
		A: Pt needs preoperative and postoperative education.
		P: Teach pt about events before and after surgery, I.V. insertion; teach about the need for coughing and deep breathing, moving frequently in bed, and early ambulation after surgery. Explain why these are important. Evaluate pt's understanding and response to the teaching, and document. ———— Ann Davis, RN

Number each problem for easy reference.

Progress notes are in SOAPIE format.

- Assessments and interventions often apply to more than one problem, so documentation of these findings is repetitious, especially with the SOAPIE format. This repetition makes documentation time-consuming to perform and read.
- The format emphasizes problems, so routine care may be left undocumented unless flow sheets are used.
- The format doesn't work well in settings with rapid patient turnover, such as a postanesthesia care unit, a short procedure unit, or an emergency department.
- Problems may arise if caregivers don't keep the problem list current or if they're confused about which problems to list.
- Considerable time and cost are needed to train people to use the SOAP, SOAPIE, and SOAPIER method.

PIE system

The problem-intervention-evaluation (PIE) system organizes information according to patients' problems and was devised to simplify the documentation process. This system requires you to keep a daily patient assessment flow sheet and to write structured progress notes. Integrating the care plan into the nurses' progress notes eliminates the need for a separate care plan. The idea is to provide a concise, efficient record of patient care that has a nursing focus. (See *Easy as PIE*, page 70.)

Using the PIE system

To use the PIE system, first assess the patient and document your findings on a daily patient assessment flow sheet.

Pieces of PIE

The daily assessment flow sheet lists defined assessment terms under major categories (such as respiration) along with routine care and monitoring measures (such as providing ventilation and monitoring breath sounds). The flow sheet generally includes space to record pertinent treatments.

On the flow sheet, initial only the assessment terms that apply to your patient and mark abnormal findings with an asterisk. Record detailed information in your progress notes.

Next, chart:
1. the patient's problems
2. your interventions
3. your evaluations of the patient's responses.

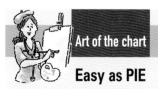

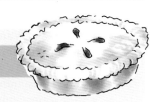

Art of the chart

Easy as PIE

This sample chart shows how to write progress notes using the problem-intervention-evaluation (PIE) system.

Date	Time	Notes
2/20/2017	1300	P#1: Sudden onset of generalized itching and hives
		IP#1: Note extent of symptoms; take VS; assess breath sounds for wheezing. Notify practitioner immediately. Administer medications as ordered. Reassure pt.
		EP#1: Symptoms abate; pt maintains adequate respiratory and hemodynamic status; pt verbalized understanding of treatments and need to report further symptoms. —————————— Mary Smith, RN
2/20/2017	1300	P#2: Ineffective breathing pattern related to possible allergic reaction.
		IP#2: Take VS frequently and monitor breath sounds and pulse oximetry. Notify practitioner for abnormal findings. Give medications as ordered. Administer oxygen by nasal cannula as ordered. Teach pt signs of respiratory distress and the need to report these immediately. —————— Mary Smith, RN
		EP#2: Pt has no wheezing or dyspnea; pt verbalized understanding of need to notify nurse of changes in breathing patterns. —————— Mary Smith, RN

[Callout: This stands for evaluation of problem # 1.]

Problem

After performing and documenting an initial assessment, use the collected data to identify pertinent nursing diagnoses. These form the *problem* piece of PIE. Use the list of nursing diagnoses accepted by your facility, which usually corresponds to the diagnoses approved by NANDA International.

Got a problem with that?

If you can't find a nursing diagnosis on an approved list, write the problem statement yourself using accepted criteria. Make sure you don't use medical diagnoses.

Keeping track

In the progress notes, document all nursing diagnoses or problems, labeling each as *P* and numbering it. For example, the first nursing diagnosis is labeled *P#1*. This way, you can later refer to a specific problem by its label only, without having to redocument the problem statement. Some facilities also use a separate problem-list form to keep a convenient running account of the nursing diagnoses for each patient.

[Speech bubble: Number each problem for future reference.]

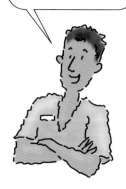

Intervention

To chart the *intervention* piece of PIE, document the nursing interventions provided for each nursing diagnosis. Write them on the progress sheet, labeling each as *I* and assigning the appropriate problem number. For example, to refer to an intervention for the first nursing diagnosis, write *IP#1*.

Evaluation

After documenting your interventions, document the patient's responses in your progress notes. These form the *evaluation* piece of PIE. Use the label *E* followed by the assigned problem number. For example, to identify each evaluation write *EP#1*.

Reevaluate and review

Make sure that you or another nurse evaluates each problem at least once every 12 hours. After every shift, review the notes from the previous 24 hours to identify the patient's current problems and responses to interventions.

Document continuing problems daily, along with relevant interventions and evaluations. Once resolved and documented as such, a problem doesn't require further documentation.

Reasons to give PIE a try

The PIE format has many attractive features, including:
- ensuring that your documentation includes all the necessary pieces: nursing diagnoses (problems), related interventions, and evaluations
- providing ongoing documentation of current problems
- encouraging you to meet The Joint Commission requirements by providing an organized framework for your thoughts and writing
- simplifying documentation by combining the care plan and progress notes and using the flow sheet for assessment and patient care data
- improving the quality of your progress notes by highlighting interventions and requiring a written evaluation of the patient's response to them.

Problems with PIE

Don't take a "pie-in-the-sky" attitude to this documentation system. Here's why:
- Staff members may need in-depth training before they can use it properly.
- There is no formal care plan, so the nurse needs to read the notes to determine problems and interventions before starting care.
- It requires you to reevaluate each problem once every shift, which is time-consuming, usually unnecessary for every problem, and leads to repetitive entries.

- It omits documentation of the planning step in the nursing process. This step, which addresses expected outcomes, is essential in evaluating the patient's responses.
- It doesn't incorporate multidisciplinary documentation.
- It isn't suitable for long-term care patients.

FOCUS (F–DAR) system

Nurses who found the SOAP format awkward developed the FOCUS (F-DAR) system of documentation. FOCUS (F-DAR) is a systematic approach to documentation that organizes patient-centered topics, or *foci* in order to make the patient, or patient concerns, the focus of care. It encourages you to use assessment data to evaluate these concerns. FOCUS (F-DAR) documentation works best in acute care settings and on units where the same care and procedures are repeated frequently. It is organized by D (data), A (action), and R (response).

Coming into FOCUS (F–DAR)

To implement FOCUS (F-DAR) documentation, you use a progress sheet with columns for the date, time, focus, and progress notes. You can identify the foci by reviewing your assessment data. (See *Focus on FOCUS (F-DAR) documentation*, page 73.)

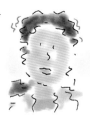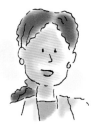

With this system of documentation, you typically write each focus as a nursing diagnosis, such as *Risk for infection* or *Deficient fluid volume*. However, the focus also may refer to:
- sign or symptom—such as purulent drainage or chest pain
- patient behavior—such as an inability to ambulate
- special need—such as a discharge or education need
- acute change in the patient's condition—such as loss of consciousness or increase in blood pressure
- significant event—such as surgery.

Writing FOCUS (F–DAR) progress notes

In the progress notes column, identify and divide the information into three categories:
1. data (D), which includes subjective and objective information describing the focus
2. action (A), which includes immediate and future nursing interventions based on your assessment of the patient's condition as well as changes to the care plan as necessary, based on your evaluation
3. response (R), which describes the patient's response to nursing or medical care.

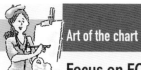

Art of the chart

Focus on FOCUS (F-DAR) documentation

The chart below is an example of progress notes using the FOCUS (F-DAR) system.

> Progress notes are divided into data, action, and response.

Date	Time	Focus	Progress notes
2/3/2017	1000	Deficient	D: Pt states she does not understand what her diagnosis means.
		knowledge	A: Illness explained to pt according to her level of
		R/T	understanding. Pt taught symptoms she may expect and why
		diagnosis	she is having current symptoms. Treatments and procedures
			explained. Questions answered. Pt encouraged to verbalize
			need for further instruction or information.
			R: Pt verbalized better understanding of her illness.
			———————————————— Donna Jones, RN
2/3/2017	1000	Risk for	D: Pt states her period just began and she is passing a large
		deficient	amount of clots.
		fluid	A: Amount of bleeding assessed. Pt saturated 2 sanitary napkins
		volume	in the past hour, currently large amount of bright red clots
			noted. BP 114/70 P 98 RR 20. Pt status reported to Dr. T. Smith.
			Orders received. 20G I.V. catheter inserted labs drawn;
			1,000 ml NSS hung, macro tubing, at 100 ml per hr. Pt
			tolerated procedures well. Will continue to monitor vital signs
			and bleeding. Pt taught how to assess amount of vaginal drainage.
			R: Pt verbalizes correct amount of drainage and type. Pt
			understands procedures. ——————— Donna Jones, RN
2/3/2017	1000	Anxiety	D: Pt states, "I'm afraid of all this blood."
			A: Emotional support provided. Encouraged verbalization.
			Explanations given regarding treatments and procedures.
			Family in to provide support.
			R: Pt observed talking and laughing with family. States she
			feels less anxious. ——————— Donna Jones, RN

> This focus is written as a nursing diagnosis.

> The foci zoom in on the topics of major concern.

Lights, camera, data, action, response!

Using all three categories guarantees complete documentation based on the nursing process. Be sure to record routine nursing tasks and assessment data on your flow sheets and checklists.

DAR–e to succeed?

FOCUS (F-DAR) documentation has several strong points:

- It's flexible enough to adapt to any clinical setting.
- It centers on the nursing process, and the data-action-response format encourages you to record in a process-oriented way.
- Information on a specific problem is easy to find because the FOCUS (F-DAR) statement is separate from the progress note. This promotes communication between health care team members.
- It encourages regular documentation of patient responses to nursing and medical care and ensures adherence to The Joint Commission requirements.
- You can use this format to document many topics in addition to those on the problem list or care plan.
- It helps you organize your thoughts and document succinctly and precisely.
- It helps you identify areas in the care plan that need revising as you document each entry.

FOCUS (F–DAR) downers

FOCUS (F-DAR) documentation also has weaknesses:

- Staff members, especially those who are more familiar with other systems, may need in-depth training before they can use it effectively.
- You have to use many flow sheets and checklists, which can cause inconsistent documentation and problems tracking a patient's problems.
- If you forget to include the patient's response to interventions, FOCUS (F-DAR) documentation resembles a long narrative, like that seen in progress notes.

Charting by exception

The system called "charting by exception" (CBE) was designed to eliminate lengthy and repetitive notes, poorly organized information, difficult-to-retrieve data, errors of omission, and other long-standing documentation problems. To avoid these pitfalls, the CBE format radically departs from traditional systems by requiring documentation of significant or abnormal findings only.

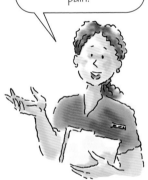

The patient's condition is unchanged, EXCEPT for reporting less pain!

CBE guidelines

To use CBE effectively, you must adhere to established guidelines for nursing assessments and interventions and follow written standards of practice that identify the nurse's basic responsibilities.

Document deviations

Guidelines for a "normal" assessment of each body system are provided as defined by your facility. (See "Defining normal parameters.") Having the "normal" findings clearly and concisely written eliminates the need to chart on acceptable findings; all you document are deviations from the guidelines.

Defining normal parameters

For facilities that utilize a "CBE" documentation system, assessment findings that are considered "normal" are usually defined and available to view while charting. Assessment findings that do not fit into the "normal" findings are what the nurse documents. This listing identifies "normal" neurologic assessment findings:
- alert & oriented ×4
- pupils equal and reactive
- clear speech
- follows commands
- denies headache
- facial symmetry intact
- no c/o numbness or tingling or sensation loss
- moves extremities purposefully, with equal strength
- no seizure activity

Get your guidelines here

Guidelines for nursing interventions used in the CBE system come from these sources:
- *nursing diagnosis–based standardized care plans*, which identify patient problems, desired outcomes, and interventions
- *patient care guidelines*, which are standardized intervention plans created for specific patients, such as those with a nursing diagnosis of *Acute pain* or *Chronic pain*, that outline the nursing interventions, treatments, and time frames for repeated assessments
- *practitioner's orders*, which are prescribed medical interventions, such as *Assist with ambulation three times daily*
- *incidental orders*, which are usually one-time, miscellaneous nursing or medical orders or interdependent interventions related to a protocol or a piece of equipment, such as *Discontinue nasogastric tube*
- *standards of nursing practice*, which define the acceptable level of routine nursing care for all patients and may describe the essential

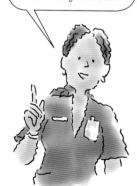

Guidelines for flying straight with the CBE system come from many sources.

aspects of nursing practice for a specific unit or for all clinical areas, such as *Vital signs every 4 hours*. Additionally, facilities define normal assessment findings as identified within the documentation system, so abnormal findings are more easily identified.

CBE format

The CBE format includes a standardized care plan based on the nursing diagnosis and several types of flow sheets, which can be individualized by each facility. These flow sheets include:
- nursing and medical order flow sheets
- assessment flow sheets
- I.V. therapy flow sheets
- graphic forms for vital sign documentation
- patient-teaching records
- patient discharge notes.

Making progress?

Sometimes, you may need to supplement your CBE documentation by using nurses' progress notes.

Standardized care plans

When using the CBE format for documentation, you utilize a standardized care plan for each nursing diagnosis. (See chapter 3, Care plans.)

Fill in the blanks

Standardized care plans provide the ability to individualize them as needed. For example, include expected outcomes and major revisions in your care plan.

Nursing flow sheets

Use nursing flow sheets to document your assessments and interventions.

The top part of the flow sheet contains the information regarding assessments and interventions, per practitioner order or facility protocol. (See *Using a nursing flow sheet*, page 77.)

Checks, asterisks, and arrows

In addition to the abbreviations, use these symbols when you record care on flow sheets:
- a check mark (✔) to indicate a completed medical order or nursing assessment with no abnormal findings
- an asterisk (✱) to indicate an abnormal finding on an assessment or an abnormal response to an intervention requiring further documentation

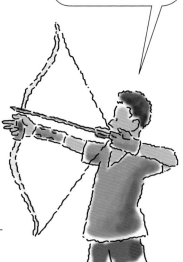

In CBE, an arrow indicates that the patient's status hasn't changed.

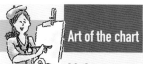

Using a nursing flow sheet

NURSING FLOW SHEET

Date 1/22/17	1900–0700	0700–1900
Respiratory		
Breath sounds	clear 2330 PW	clear 1600 MLF
Treatments/results	————	————
Cough/results	————	————
O₂ therapy	Nasal cannula @ 2 L/min PW	Nasal cannula @ 2 L/min MLF
Cardiac		
Chest pain	s̄ PW	s̄ MLF
Heart sounds	Normal S₁ and S₂ PW	Normal S1 and S2 MLF
Telemetry	N/A	N/A
Pain		
Type and location	Ⓛ flank 0400 PW	Ⓛ flank 0400 MLF
Intervention	Meperidine 0415 PW	Meperidine 1615 MLF
Pt. response	Improved from #9 to #3 in 1/2 hr PW	Complete relief in hr MLF
Nutrition		
Type	————	Regular MLF
Toleration %	————	80% MLF
Supplement	————	————
Elimination		
Stool appearance	s̄ PW	s̄ soft dark brown MLF
Enema	N/A	N/A
Results	————	————
Bowel sounds	Present all quadrants 2330 PW	Hyperactive all quadrants 1600 MLF
Urine appearance	Clear, amber 0400 PW	
Indwelling urinary catheter	N/A	N/A
Catheter irrigations	————	————

- an arrow (➔) to indicate that the patient's status hasn't changed since the previous entry.

After completing an assessment, compare your findings with the printed guidelines on the back of the form. If a finding is within normal parameters, place a check mark in the appropriate box. If a finding isn't within the normal range, put an asterisk in the box. Then explain your findings in the comment section on the form or electronic screen.

Note normalcy

An assessment finding that isn't defined in the guidelines may be normal for a particular patient. For example, unclear speech may be normal in a patient with a long-standing tracheostomy. Reference this type of note by nursing diagnosis number. If the patient's condition hasn't changed from the last assessment, draw a horizontal arrow from the previous category box to the current one.

Make more marks

Document interventions similarly. Use a check mark to indicate a completed intervention and an expected patient response. Indicate significant findings or abnormal patient responses with an asterisk and write an explanation in the comment section. When the patient's response is unchanged, use an arrow.

If using a paper form, after you document an entire column in the assessments and interventions section, initial it at the bottom. Also initial all your entries in the comment section and sign the form at the bottom of the page. Electronic documentation will supply an electronic signature related to your log in.

Care-ful combinations

Some facilities use a special nursing care flow sheet that combines all the necessary forms, such as the graphic record, the daily activities checklist, and the patient care assessment section. (See *It flows together: Using a combined nursing care flow sheet*, page 79.)

Graphic form

The graphic form section of a flow sheet is used to document trends in the patient's vital signs, weight, intake and output, and stool, urination, appetite, and activity levels.

More checks and asterisks

As with the nursing flow sheet, use check marks to indicate expected findings and asterisks to indicate abnormal ones. Record information about abnormalities in the nurses' progress notes or on the nursing flow sheet in the designated area for comments.

In the box labeled "routine standards," check off the established nursing care interventions you performed such as providing hygiene.

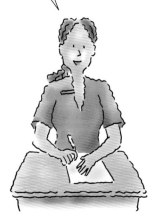

If your patient has multiple learning needs, you can use more than one form.

(Text continues on page 82.)

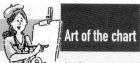

Art of the chart

It flows together: Using a combined nursing care flow sheet

This sample shows a portion of a nursing care flow sheet that combines a graphic record, a daily nursing care activities checklist, and a patient care assessment form.

Name _____ Maureen Gallen _____

> The graphic record makes it easy to spot trends.

Date		2/29/2017										
Hour		0700	0800	0900	1000	1100	1200	1300	1400	1500	1600	1700	1800

Temperature

°C	°F
40.6	105
40	104
39.4	103
38.9	102
37.8	100
37.2	99
36.7	98
36.1	97
35.6	96

		0700	0800	0900	1000	1100	1200	1300	1400	1500	1600	1700	1800
Pulse		84	80	82	78	76	78	78	82	84	82	80	78
Respiration		16	20	20	22	24	24	18	20	22	20	18	24
BP	Lying												
	Sitting	136/82	130/80	126/74	132/82	132/80	140/82	136/74	130/70	138/78	140/80	132/78	136/76
	Standing												
Intake	Oral		240					360					120
	Tube												
	I.V.												
	Blood												
8-hour total		—	—	—	—	—	—	—	—	600	—	—	—
Output			400				450						
Other													
8-hour total		—	—	—	—	—	—	—	—	850	—	—	—
Teaching		dressing changes, s/s of infection											

Signature		Mary Murphy, RN		Ann Burns, RN	
		0700 - 1900		1900 - 0700	

(continued)

It flows together: Using a combined nursing care flow sheet (continued)

This section enables efficient documentation of daily activities.

Hour		0700	0800	0900	1000	1100	1200	1300	1400	1500	1600	1700
ACTIVITY	Bed rest	MM	→						→	AB	→	→
	OOB											
	Ambulate (assist)											
	Ambulatory											
	Sleeping											
	Bathroom privileges											
	HOB elevated	MM	→						→	AB	→	→
	Cough, deep-breathe, turn		MM								AB	
	ROM Active / Passive		MM								AB	
HYGIENE	Bath		MM									
	Shave		MM									
	Oral		MM									
	Skin care											
	Peri care											
NUTRITION	Diet	House										
	% eating			75%			60%					75%
	Feeding											
	Supplemental											
	S-Self, A-Assist, F-Feed		A				A					A
BLADDER	Catheter	indwelling urinary #18 Fr.										
	Incontinent											
	Voiding	clear, yellow urine										
	Intermittent catheter											
BOWEL	Stools (occult blood + or −)											
	Incontinent											
	Normal	large formed brown stool										
	Enema											
SPECIAL TREATMENTS	Special mattress	Low-pressure airflow mattress applied 0900										
	Special bed											
	Heel and elbow pads											
	Antiembolism stockings											
	Traction: + = on, − = off											
	Isolation type											

It flows together: Using a combined nursing care flow sheet (continued)

ASSESSMENT FINDINGS

Findings marked by an asterisk must be documented.

KEY: ✓ = normal findings
✱ = significant findings

	Day	Night	
Neurologic	✱ MM		0800 Limited ROM ⓛ shoulder. Pt. states, "I have arthritis and my shoulder is always stiff."
Cardiovascular	✓ MM		
Respiratory	✱ MM		1800 Shallow breathing with poor inspiratory effort at 1700.
GI	✓ MM		
Genitourinary	✓ MM		
Surgical dressing and incision	✱ MM		0930 Incision reddened; dime-sized area of serous sanguineous drainage on old dressing
Skin integrity	✓ MM		
Psychosocial	✓ MM		
Educational	✱ MM		0945 Taught pt incisional care and dressing change, and s/s of infection. Pt. able to return demonstration of incisional care.
Peripheral vascular	✓ MM		

(continued)

It flows together: Using a combined nursing care flow sheet *(continued)*

NORMAL ASSESSMENT FINDINGS

Neurologic assessment:
* Alert and oriented to time, place, and person.
* Speech clear and understandable.
* Memory intact.
* Behavior appropriate to situation and accommodation.
* Active range of motion (ROM) of all extremities, symmetrically equal strength.
* No paresthesia.

Cardiovascular assessment:
* Regular apical pulse.
* Palpable bilateral peripheral pulses.
* No peripheral edema.
* No calf tenderness.

Pulmonary assessment:
* Resting respirations 10 to 20 per minute, quiet and regular.
* Clear sputum.
* Pink nail beds and mucous membranes.

Gastrointestinal assessment:
* Abdomen soft and nondistended.
* Tolerates prescribed diet without nausea or vomiting.
* Bowel movements within own normal pattern and consistency (as described in Patient Profile).

Genitourinary assessment:
* No indwelling catheter in use.
* Urinates without pain.
* Undistended bladder after urination.
* Urine is clear, yellow to amber color.

Surgical dressing and incision assessment:
* Dressing dry and intact.
* No evidence of redness, increased temperature, or tenderness in surrounding tissue.
* Sutures, staples, or adhesive strips intact.
* Wound edges well-approximated.
* No drainage present.

Skin integrity assessment:
* Skin color normal.
* Skin warm, dry, and intact.
* Moist mucous membranes.

Psychosocial assessment:
* Interacts and communicates in an appropriate manner with others (family, significant others, health care personnel).

Educational assessment:
* Patient or significant others communicate understanding of the patient's health status, care plan, and expected response.
* Patient or significant others demonstrate ability to perform health-related procedures and behaviors as taught.
* Items taught and expected performance must be specifically described in Significant Findings Section.

Peripheral vascular assessment:
* Affected extremity is pink, warm, and movable within average ROM.
* Capillary refill time less than 3 seconds.
* Peripheral pulses palpable.
* No edema, sensation intact without numbness or paresthesia.
* No pain on passive stretch.

Don't rewrite these standards as orders on the nursing and medical order flow sheet. Refer to the guidelines on the back of the graphic form for complete instructions.

Patient-teaching record

Use the patient-teaching form (or section) to identify the information, psychomotor skills, and social or behavioral measures that your patient or the patient's caregiver must learn by a set goal date. Document understanding of the teaching provided as well as follow-up teaching that is needed.

It's exception-all

The CBE format has several important benefits:
* It eliminates documentation of routine care through the use of nursing care standards. This stops redundancies and clearly identifies abnormal data. It may also save time.

- CBE is easily adapted to documentation on care pathway.
- Information that has already been recorded isn't repeated. For instance, you don't have to write a long entry each time you assess a patient whose condition has stayed the same.
- The use of well-defined guidelines and standards of care promotes uniform nursing practice.
- The flow sheets let you track trends easily.
- Guidelines are available for ready reference of what is considered acceptable assessment findings for "normal." Abnormal findings are documented to help you quickly pinpoint significant changes and trends in a patient's condition.
- Patient data are immediately documented on the permanent record. Because you don't need to keep temporary notes and then transcribe them in the patient's chart later, all caregivers always have access to the most current data, which decreases documentation time.
- Assessments are standardized, so all caregivers evaluate and document findings consistently.
- All flow sheets are kept at the patient's bedside, where they serve as a ready reference. This encourages immediate documentation.

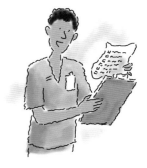

With CBE, I don't waste time documenting routine care.

CBE shortcomings

Nothing is perfect, including the CBE system. Here are the drawbacks:
- The development of clear guidelines and standards of care is time-consuming. For legal reasons, these guidelines and standards must be written and understood by all nurses before the system can be implemented.
- This system takes a long time for people to learn, accept, and use correctly and consistently.
- Duplicate documentation occurs with CBE; nursing diagnoses on a problem list are also written on the care plan.
- A lack of detail may create a legal problem or may compromise patient safety as it may fail to alert other health care members of a problem or complication accurately.
- Narrative notes and evaluations of patients' responses may be brief and sketchy in facilities that use multiple forms instead of one combination form.
- This system was developed for RNs. Before LPNs can use it, it must be evaluated and modified to meet their scope of practice.

Electronic health record

Whenever a patient enters a health care facility—whether it's a hospital, nursing home, or practitioner's office—a lot of information about that patient is obtained, documented, and processed. This information must be documented so that it's easily retrievable as well as meaningful and useful to other health care providers. The EHR, also known as the electronic medical record (EMR), is the standard in over 90% of health care facilities as it is designed to retain patient information more efficiently and to transfer patient information easily between facilities.

Consider me part of the health care team!

Information station

The EHR consists of a complex, interconnected set of software applications that process and transport data that are input by the health care team. The EHR categorizes the patient's data and stores the patient's health care history, including inpatient and outpatient records from various facilities. This information helps guide the health care team in providing care and identifying patient education needs.

Multitasker

In addition to helping with patient needs, the EHR can assist with:
- nurse-management reports
- patient classification data
- federal and state licensure and accreditation surveys
- research data.

The upside

The advantages of an EHR include:
- improved standardized documentation
- higher quality of clinical information within the medical record
- quick access to patient information across all departments as well as other health care institutions
- reduction in redundant documentation
- improved legibility
- ability to document patient information at the bedside
- promotes paperless system
- potential time saver.

Can't make heads or tails of a practitioner's written orders? An electronic health record can help clear things up!

The downside

EHR's also have their disadvantages:
- Computer crashes or breakdowns can make patient information temporarily unavailable.
- Computer downtime for system updates makes information unavailable for a short period each day.
- Conversion to EHR system, equipment maintenance, software updates, and training of staff is costly.
- Breaches in patient confidentiality may occur.

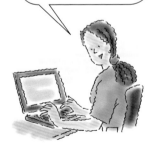

Using an EHR

For use of an EHR, most health care facilities have a mainframe computer as well as personal computers or terminals at workstations throughout the facility. These terminals provide quick access to vital information and allow staff to easily enter patient care orders. Some facilities also have bedside terminals or computers on wheels that make data even more accessible or documentation easier because it can be completed at the bedside.

Mum's the word

Each team member is assigned an individual username and password. Confidentiality laws and guidelines prohibit the sharing of computer access. Your password is a legal electronic signature that's individual to you. It is imperative to log off when leaving a computer terminal. Staying logged in allows someone else access to patient information or documentation using your name.

Starting the record

When a patient is admitted into the facility, patient information regarding name, age, address, and insurance is entered into the computer and an account number and medical record number is then assigned. This begins the patient's computerized record.

Individual access

With computerized documentation, different members of the health care team can have access to different levels of patient information. For example, a dietitian who logs into the patient record with a username and password may see dietary orders but not physical therapy orders. A charge nurse on a unit typically has access to more patient information than a bedside nurse because of the need to oversee different aspects of patient care. When used appropriately, the differentiation in access levels help to maintain a patient's privacy. (See *Maintaining patient confidentiality*, page 86.)

Practitioner's use

After the patient's registered in the computer, a practitioner can log into the specific version of the system called *computerized physician order entry* (CPOE) to enter orders that are appropriate for the patient, either from an established order set or as individual orders. Then the orders will be visible to the nursing staff so they can be verified and transmitted to the appropriate departments, such as radiology or the laboratory department. Some programs have medication orders transmit to the pharmacy as well as to the nursing staff for quicker treatment.

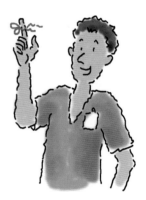

Remember, your password is a legal electronic signature. Don't allow anyone else to use it.

Maintaining patient confidentiality

The American Nurses Association and the American Records Association offer these guidelines for maintaining confidentiality of the electronic health record (EHR).

Never share
Never give your personal password or computer code to anyone—including another nurse in the unit, a nurse serving temporarily in the unit, or a practitioner. Your health care facility can issue a short-term password that allows infrequent users to access certain records.

Log off
After you log on to a computer terminal, don't leave the terminal unattended. Although some computer systems have a timing device that automatically logs off the user after an idle period, you should develop the habit of logging off the system before leaving the terminal.

Don't display
Don't leave information about a patient displayed on a monitor where others can see it. Also, don't leave print versions or excerpts of the medical record unattended.

Help for managing meds

Because the EHR allows for direct order transmittal, it cuts down on medication errors by eliminating order transcription errors, especially related to legibility. It also alerts the health care team to patient allergies. Additionally, the system's medication order screens typically provide the practitioner with choices of dosages and administration routes, which can help prevent dosing errors.

Ready, set, document

Once a patient is available in the electronic system, you can enter assessment information, create or update the care plan or progress notes, view test results or notations made by other members of the multidisciplinary team, and view practitioners orders.

Fast and functional

Typically, EHRs allow health care providers to retrieve information more quickly than traditional documentation systems do. Most electronic systems allow you to print a patient Kardex or worklist each shift that contains information and interventions to guide your care. (See *Computer-generated Kardex*, page 87.)

Follow protocol

Be sure to follow your facility's protocol and systems direction for correcting errors in the EHR. Computer entries are part of the

I can't find anything in this mess! Get me a computerized documentation system STAT!

(Text continues on page 89.)

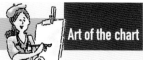

Art of the chart

Computer-generated Kardex

The computer-generated Kardex contains vital information to help guide your nursing care throughout your shift. It may be necessary to print out a new Kardex at various times throughout your shift, so new practitioner's orders are reflected.

Medical ICU—4321 Patient Care Hospital   PAGE 01
03/14/2017   07:00   **PATIENT KARDEX**

WILLIAMS, HENRY   68   MWMC
MR#: 5555555   DOB 10/26/40   MICU   302
FIN#: 1010101010   Admitted: 03/12/2017
DR: Daniel Smith   Service: Internal Medicine

Summary: 03/14/2017 0700-1900

ALLERGIES AND CODE STATUS:
03/12/2017   MED ALLERGY: NO KNOWN DRUG ALLERGY   NO INTUBATION

PATIENT INFORMATION:
03/12/2017   Admit Dx: TIA
03/13/2017   Final Dx: Stroke
03/12/2017   Patient condition: Fair
03/13/2017   Clinical guideline: Stroke
03/12/2017   Language: English
03/12/2017   PMH: No problems—respiratory, HTN, No problems—GI, No problems—GU, Type 2 diabetes, No problems—skin, No problems—blood, No problems—musculoskeletal, No problems—psych, No problems—hearing, glasses, cholecystectomy 1982, Tobacco use: denies, Alcohol use: current, 1 beer a day, Illicit drug use: denies, Immunizations: Flu vaccine: 2008
03/12/2017   Living will: yes, on chart
03/12/2017   Durable power of attorney: yes, Name of DPOA: June Smith, Phone number 9875551234
03/12/2017   Organ donor: yes, card on chart

CONSULTS:
03/12/2017   Consult Westside Neurological Associates to see patient regarding flaccid left side and expressive aphasia

ISF NOTES:
03/12/2017   Care plan: General care of the adult
03/12/2017   Nursing protocol: Falls prevention
03/12/2017   Nursing protocol: Skin breakdown (prevention)
03/12/2017   Goal: Patient will tolerate a progressive increase in activity level.

NURSE COMMUNICATIONS:
03/12/2017   I.V. site—RA2, #20 inserted, restart on 03/15/2017   CONTINUED

(continued)

Computer-generated Kardex *(continued)*

```
                                                              PAGE 02
03/14/2017        07:00                    PATIENT KARDEX
WILLIAMS, HENRY    68                      MWMC
MR#: 5555555       DOB 10/26/40   MICU            302
FIN#: 1010101010             Admitted: 03/12/2017
DR: Daniel Smith        Service: Internal Medicine
Summary: 03/14/2017  0700-1900
```

ALL CURRENT MEDICAL ORDERS

Doctor to nurse orders:

03/12/2017	Blood cultures × 2 if temperature greater than 101° F, Nurse please enter as a secondary order, when necessary.
03/12/2017	Cardiology: ECG 12 lead Stat, prn chest pain, Nurse please enter as a secondary order, when necessary.
03/12/2017	Sequential compression therapy: Patient to wear continuously while in bed.
03/12/2017	Indwelling urinary catheter to urometer, measure output q 1 hour, notify MD if urine output less than 30 ml in one hour or greater than 300 ml in 2 hours.
03/12/2017	Notify MD for SBP greater than 180 mm Hg or less than 110 mm Hg
03/12/2017	Notify MD for change in mental status
03/12/2017	Accucheck q 6 hours

Vital sign orders:

03/12/2017	VS: q 1 hour with neurologic checks

Diet:

03/12/2017	NPO

I&O orders:

03/12/2017	Per ICU routine

Activity:

03/12/2017	Bedrest with HOB elevated 30 degrees

IVS:

03/12/2017	I.V. line—Dextrose 5% & Sodium Chloride 0.45% 1000 ml, Rate: 80 ml per hour, 2 bags

Scheduled medications:

03/12/2017	Dexamethasone 4 mg, I.V., q 6 hours
03/12/2017	Metoprolol 5 mg, I.V., q 6 hours
03/12/2017	Heparin 5,000 units, subcutaneously, q 12 hours

Miscellaneous Medications:

03/13/2017	Furosemide 40 mg, I.V., Now

PRN Medications:

03/12/2017	Acetaminophen Supp 650 mg, #1, PR, q 4 hour prn pain or temperature greater than 101° F

Laboratory:

03/14/2017	Basic metabolic panel tomorrow, collect at 05:00
03/14/2017	CBC/Diff/Plts tomorrow, collect at 05:00
03/14/2017	Cardiac troponin, tomorrow, collect at 05:00

CONTINUED

Computer-generated Kardex *(continued)*

```
                                                                    PAGE 03
03/14/2017        07:00                          PATIENT KARDEX

WILLIAMS, HENRY    68                      MWMC
MR#: 5555555       DOB 10/26/40   MICU          302
FIN#: 1010101010                  Admitted: 03/12/2017
DR: Daniel Smith                  Service: Internal Medicine

Summary: 03/14/2017  0700-1900


Radiology:
   03/12/2017    Computed tomography: CT scan of the head without contrast STAT
Ancillary:
   03/12/2017    Respiratory care: Oxygen via nasal cannula at 2 L/minute
   03/12/2017    Physical therapy: Patient evaluation and treatment         LAST PAGE
```

patient's permanent record and, as such, can't be deleted. Most systems have a special feature that allows you to correct or "undo" a documentation error. Be sure to enter the date and time the error was made and enter the correct information, if able. Although some error correction may not be easily seen, computer software will retain the information.

Types of EHR systems

Specialized nursing information systems (NISs) can increase your efficiency in all phases of documentation. (See *Electronic documentation and the nursing process*, page 90.)

Talk, touch, or click

Depending on which type of computer hardware and software your health care facility has purchased, you may access information by using your voice, a keyboard, a light pen, a touch-sensitive screen, or a mouse.

Adding your personal touch

With some systems, you can use a menu of common phrases to quickly create a narrative note. You can also elaborate on a problem or clarify flow sheet documentation in the comment section of a computerized form by entering standardized phrases or typing in comments.

Electronic documentation and the nursing process

An electronic documentation system can either stand alone or be a subsystem of a larger hospital system. Nursing information systems (NISs) can increase efficiency and accuracy in all phases of the nursing process—assessment, nursing diagnosis, planning, implementation, and evaluation—and can help nurses meet the standards established by the American Nurses Association and The Joint Commission. In addition, NISs can help nurses spend more time meeting patient needs. Consider these uses of computers in the nursing process.

Assessment

You can use the computer terminal to record admission information. As you collect data, enter additional information as prompted by the computer's software program. Enter data about the patient's health status, history, chief complaint, and other assessment factors.

Some software programs prompt you to ask specific questions and then offer pathways to gather further information. In some systems, the computer program flags assessment values that are outside the usual acceptable range to call attention to them.

Nursing diagnosis

Most current programs list standard diagnoses with associated signs and symptoms as references. However, you must still use clinical judgment to determine a nursing diagnosis for each patient. With this information, you can rapidly obtain diagnostic information. For example, the computer can generate a list of possible diagnoses for a patient with selected signs and symptoms or it may

enable you to retrieve and review the patient's records according to the nursing diagnosis.

Planning

To help nurses develop a care plan, some computer programs display recommended expected outcomes and interventions for the selected diagnosis. Computers can also track outcomes for large patient populations. You can use computers to compare large amounts of patient data, help identify outcomes the patient is likely to achieve based on individual problems and needs, and estimate the time frame for reaching outcome goals.

Implementation

You can also use the computer to record actual interventions and patient-processing information, such as transfer and discharge instructions, and to communicate this information to other departments. Computer-generated progress notes automatically sort and print out patient data—such as medication administration, treatments, and vital signs—making documentation more efficient and accurate.

Evaluation

During evaluation, you can use the computer to record and store observations, patient responses to nursing interventions, and your own evaluation statements. You may also use information from other members of the health care team to determine future actions and discharge planning. If a desired patient outcome has not been achieved, record new interventions taken to ensure desired outcomes. Then reevaluate the second set of interventions.

What's your type?

Types of computerized documentation systems include:
- specialized NISs
- nursing minimum data set (NMDS)
- nursing outcomes classification (NOC) system
- voice-activated systems.

Nursing information system

Current NIS software programs allow nurses to record nursing actions in the patient's EHR. These systems incorporate most or all of the components of the nursing process so they can meet the standards of the American Nurses Association and The Joint Commission. Furthermore, each NIS provides different features and can be customized to conform to a facility's documentation forms and formats. For example, some systems offer automated drug information, guidelines regarding facility policies and procedures, and intranet access. Other systems may provide the capability for online literature searches, which keeps the latest health care information at the nurse's fingertips.

From passive to interactive

NIS programs can manage information passively, actively, or interactively. Passive systems collect, transmit, organize, format, print, and display information that you can use to help make a decision, but they don't make that decision for you. Active systems suggest nursing diagnoses based on predefined assessment data that you enter. The most recent NIS programs take this functionality a step further, interacting with you based on the information you enter. (See *Computerized give-and-take.*)

Nursing minimum data set

The NMDS is a means of standardizing nursing information. It contains three categories of data:
1. nursing care, such as nursing diagnoses and interventions
2. patient demographics, such as the patient's name, birth date, gender, race or ethnicity, and residence
3. service elements, such as length of hospitalization.

Consistent and coded

The standardized format of the NMDS encourages consistent documentation. Data are coded, making documentation and information retrieval faster and easier. For example, NANDA International assigns numerical codes to all nursing diagnoses so they can be used with the NMDS.

Nurse's little helper

The NMDS documentation system helps you to:
- collect nursing diagnoses and intervention data, which can be used to plan patient care
- identify the nursing needs of various patient populations
- track patient outcomes

Computerized give-and-take

Most nursing information systems interact with you, prompting you with questions and suggestions about the information you enter. Ultimately, this computerized, sequential decision-making format should lead to more effective nursing care and documentation.

An interactive system requires you to enter only a brief narrative. The questions and suggestions the computer program provides make your documentation thorough and quick. The program also allows you to add or change information so that your documentation is tailored to fit your patient.

- describe nursing care received in different settings, including the patient's home
- establish accurate estimates for nursing service costs
- compare nursing trends locally, regionally, and nationally
- compare nursing data from various clinical settings, patient populations, and geographic areas
- obtain data about nursing care that may influence health care policy and decision making.

But it's always about the patient

Above all, the NMDS helps you provide better patient care. For example, examining the outcomes of various patient populations may help set realistic outcomes for an individual patient.

Nursing outcomes classification system

The NOC system provides the first comprehensive, standardized method of measuring nursing-sensitive patient outcomes. This system benefits the nursing profession by:
- allowing the comparison of patient outcomes with the outcomes of larger groups that share similar ages, diagnoses, or health care settings
- serving as an essential tool in ongoing nursing research
- including patient data-related outcomes, which in the past have been absent from computerized medical information databases.

Voice-activated systems

Some facilities have voice-activated nursing documentation systems. A voice-activated system combines a specialized knowledge base of words, phrases, and report forms with automated speech recognition technology. Voice-activated systems are most useful in departments that have a high volume of structured reports, such as operating rooms.

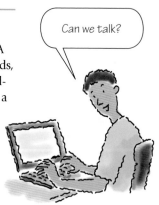

Can we talk?

Look ma, no hands!

Voice-activated systems require little or no keyboard use—you simply speak into a telephone handset and the text appears on the computer screen. You can record complete nurses' notes by simply talking.

Report support and more

In addition to report forms, the computer program includes information on the nursing process, nursing theory, and nursing standards of practice. Trigger phrases spoken by the nurse cue the system to display passages of report text and allow word-for-word dictation and editing. You can use the text displayed to design an individualized care plan or to fill in standard facility forms.

Hanging on every word

Although voice-activated systems work most efficiently with trigger phrases, word-for-word dictation and editing are also possible.

Additional system features

Depending on the system type, a computerized documentation system may provide the ability to print out patient schedules. The system may also be equipped with bar code technology.

Patient schedules

Most systems have the ability to print out schedule lists for patients. For example, you can print out a schedule of patients who require fingerstick glucose level tests. If the situation requires you to delegate the task, the list may be given to ancillary staff members. The list lets them know exactly when they're supposed to obtain the fingerstick glucose level for each patient.

Bar code technology

Bar code technology can be incorporated into computerized documentation and used for medication or blood administration. Using bar code technology increases safety regarding medication and blood delivery because it allows for specific identification of medication and blood related to the patient's identification numbers.

Medication administration

Bar code technology allows you to scan a drug's bar code and the patient's identification bracelet to help confirm the right patient, right medication, right dose, right route, and right time. Documentation of the nurse administering the medication is achieved by the nurse logging into the computer system, or scanning a personal name badge.

To be discontinued . . .

Bar code technology also helps keep track of discontinued medications. The system connects to the order-entry system, so if a practitioner discontinues a medication, it won't show up on the patient's listed medications when you scan the patient's wristband.

Sorry, wrong number

Scanning of medications also ensures that the nurse hasn't inadvertently picked the wrong medication out of the medication drawer or received the wrong medication from the pharmacy.

Streamlined service

Other advantages of bar code technology include saved time and streamlined documentation. If a patient refuses a medication, the nurse can document it immediately into the computer. At the end of the shift, the nurse-manager can print a report to identify patients who didn't receive their medications. It can also help monitor narcotic use and waste.

Blood administration

Blood administration is enhanced with bar code technology because it allows for scanning of the patient's identification and blood band, along with the blood bag codes to confirm that the blood product matches the patient's blood type, thereby decreasing the chance for incompatible blood transfusion errors. The computer prompts the nurse to follow key steps of the transfusion process to improve safety. The bar code system also removes the need for a second checker for blood administration, thereby reducing the time from collection of the blood product to actual administration.

Support provided

The Joint Commission and the Institute for Safe Medication Practices support use of medical bar code technology at the bedside. Additionally, the U.S. Food and Drug Administration's requirement that all drug makers use bar codes on medications commonly used in hospitals has led to widespread use of this system.

When computers fail

Computerized documentation makes storing and retrieving information fast and easy. But what happens when the computer system fails? Many facilities keep backup paperwork in case the computerized system fails. For this reason, you should familiarize yourself with the "down time" paper documentation forms that are available to you and follow facility protocols for completion. Documentation must be thorough—even under extreme circumstances—so make sure that you're familiar with your facility's forms and that your documentation is complete.

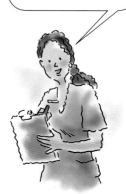

Technology is great, but it isn't perfect. You'll still need to be familiar with paper documentation in case the computer system fails.

Choosing a documentation system

Health care facilities are always striving for greater efficiency and quality of care. A top-notch documentation system can help a facility reach these goals.

Remember, documentation is examined often to make sure a facility meets the profession's minimum acceptable level of care. If efficiency and quality levels are low, your documentation system may need to be modified or replaced. (See *Does your documentation system measure up?*, page 95.)

Does your documentation system measure up?

How useful is your current documentation system? Is it incomplete, disorganized, or confusing? If so, it won't stand up to later scrutiny in case of a lawsuit or formal review or survey. To evaluate your documentation system, ask yourself the following questions. If you answer "no" to any of them, a closer evaluation of your system might be warranted.

Documenting interventions and patient progress

• Does your current system reflect the patient's progress and the interventions based on recorded evaluations? Look for records that describe the patient's progress, actual interventions, and evaluations of provided care.
• Does the record include evidence of the patient's response to nursing care? For example, does it report the effectiveness of analgesics or the patient's response to intravenous (I.V.) medications?
• Does it show that care was modified according to the patient's response to treatment? For example, does it show what action was taken if the patient tolerated only half of a prescribed tube feeding?
• Does the record note continuity of care or do unexplained gaps appear? If gaps appear, are notes entered later that document previous happenings? If late entries appear in the nurses' notes on subsequent days, do you have to check the entire record to validate care?
• Are daily activities documented? For example, do the notes include evidence that the patient is able to perform self-care or indicate the ability to independently transfer from a bed to a wheelchair?

Documenting the health care team's actions

• Does the record portray the nursing process clearly? Look for actual nursing diagnoses, written assessments, interventions, and evaluation of the patient's responses to them. Updates to the nursing diagnoses should also be apparent.
• Does the current documentation system facilitate and show communication among health care team members? Check for evidence that practitioners were notified of changes in a patient's condition and that actions reflected these communications.
• Is discharge planning clearly documented? Do the records show evidence of interdisciplinary coordination, team conferences, patient teaching, and provision of discharge instructions?
• Does the record reflect current standards of care? Does it indicate that caregivers and administrators follow facility policies and procedures? If not, does the system provide for explanations of why a policy wasn't implemented or was implemented in a different way?

Checking for clarity and comprehensiveness

• Are all portions of the record complete? Are all flow sheets, checklists, and other forms completed according to facility policy? Is medication administration accurate? If not, does the record describe why a medication wasn't given as ordered and who was informed of the omission, if necessary?
• Does the documentation make sense? Can you track the patient's care and hospital course on this record alone?

Getting better and better

Continuous quality improvement programs are mandated by the state and The Joint Commission. Committees that set up these programs choose well-defined, objective, and easily measurable indicators that help them assess the structure, process, and outcome of patient care. They also use these indicators to monitor and evaluate the contents of a patient's medical record.

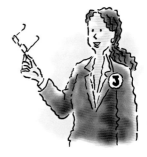

Does your documentation measure up?

Shorter hospital stays and the requirement to verify the need for supplies and equipment have placed greater emphasis on nursing documentation as a yardstick for measuring the quality of patient care and determining if it was required and provided.

To verify that treatment was required and provided or that medical tests and supplies were used, the insurers (also called *third-party payers*) review nursing documentation carefully. As a result, nurses now need to document more information than ever before, including every procedure or treatment performed.

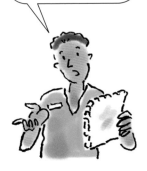

What documentation system should I use? Let's see, I need to consider the type of care my facility provides.

Are you committed? Serve on a committee . . .

When changes are called for, you may be asked to participate in a committee that evaluates your facility documentation system, or aspects of the system to determine if it needs revision or total overhaul. Before committing to a totally new system, the facility administrators should discuss the possibility of revising the current system. This may be easier and less costly than switching to a new system, changing the way information is collected, entered, and retrieved, and creating the need for staff training. (See *To change or not to change*.)

If your facility decides to switch to a new documentation system, consider the type of care that's provided at your facility. For example, some systems work better in acute care than in long-term care settings.

If a new documentation system is selected, staff will require plenty of training and the development of "experts" in the system to help with transition to a new way to document care. The system may be initiated on one unit at a time to make the transition easier.

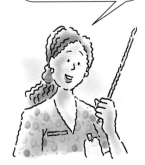

Don't miss the review of documentation systems on the next page.

To change or not to change

Whether you're selecting a new documentation system or modifying an existing one, ponder the following questions:
- What are the specific positive features of our current documentation system?
- What are the specific problems or limitations of our current system? How can they be resolved?
- How much time will we need to develop a new system, educate the staff, and implement the changes?
- Will a new system be cost-effective?
- How will changing the documentation system affect other members of the health care team, including the business office staff and medical staff?
- How will we handle resistance to the proposed changes?

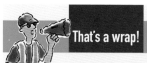

That's a wrap!

Review of documentation systems

Traditional narrative
- Flexible, easy-to-learn system that keeps notes in chronologic order, making them accessible, but may be time-consuming, repetitive, and difficult to read and understand
- Requires the nurse to be descriptive and specific about patient progress

Problem-oriented medical record
- Problem-oriented medical record (POMR) system, which uses multidisciplinary progress notes and a four-part format (database, problem list, initial plan, progress notes)
- Works well in acute and long-term care settings
- Facilitates communication between disciplines, which results in continuity of care
- Organization by problem makes assessments and interventions difficult to follow and allows routine care to go undocumented.

Problem-intervention-evaluation
- Problem-intervention-evaluation (PIE) system that isn't multidisciplinary and uses daily assessment flow sheets and nursing-focused progress notes, eliminating the need for a separate care plan
- Ensures that notes have necessary information: problems, interventions, and evaluation of the patient's response
- Elimination of planning step makes tracking patient evaluation difficult

FOCUS (F-DAR)
- Adaptable system that typically uses a nursing diagnosis–based focus to organize information

- Use of three categories (data, action, response) guarantees complete documentation that's based on the nursing process.
- Use of many flow sheets can cause inconsistent documentation and problems tracking patient complications.

Charting by exception
- Charting by exception (CBE) system that was designed to eliminate repetitive notes, poor organization, and other documentation problems by requiring that only significant or abnormal findings be documented
- Requires the nurse to adhere to established guidelines and follow written standards of practice
- Includes a standardized care plan based on the nursing diagnosis and several types of flow sheets (nursing and medical order flow sheets, graphic form, patient-teaching record, patient discharge note)

Electronic health record
- Improves standardized documentation by incorporating higher quality clinical information within the medical record
- Provides quick access to patient information across all departments
- Results in a reduction in redundant documentation as well as improved legibility in practitioner orders, decreasing errors in transmission, as well as ability to review progress notes more easily
- Provides ability to print patient schedules or Kardexes
- Can incorporate bar code technology to improve safety of drug and blood administration

Suggested references

Newton, L., and Schleppy, L. "DAR Charting Guidelines," 2010. Available: http://hfsc .org/sites/default/files/student_orientation/DAR_Charting_Guidelines.pdf.

Nursing Service Organization. "Charting by Exception: The Legal Risks," n.d. Available: https://www.nso.com/Learning/Artifacts/Articles/Charting-by-exception-the -legal-risks.

Nursing Times. "Reducing Errors in Blood Transfusion with Barcodes," 2015. Available: https://www.nursingtimes.net/clinical-archive/patient-safety/reducing-errors -in-blood-transfusion-with-barcodes/5083958.article.

Sittig, D.F., and Singh, H. "Assessing the Safety of Electronic Health Records: What Have We Learned?" 2017. Available: https://psnet.ahrq.gov/perspectives /perspective/233/assessing-the-safety-of-electronic-health-records-what-have -we-learned.

Vera, M. "Focus Charting (F-DAR): How to Do Focus Charting or F-DAR," 2011. Available: https://nurseslabs.com/focus-charting-f-dar-how-to/.

Chapter 5

Enhancing your documentation

Just the facts

In this chapter, you'll learn:

- ◆ seven rules of clear documentation and how to follow them
- ◆ different types of practitioner's orders and how to clarify them
- ◆ the nurse's role in documenting practitioner's orders.

A look at expert documentation

Documenting like a pro can be simple, but it requires adherence to seven fundamental rules:

1. Document care completely, concisely, and accurately.
2. Record observations objectively.
3. Document information promptly. Include the date and time of events.
4. Write legibly.
5. Use approved abbreviations.
6. Use the proper technique to correct documentation errors.
7. Sign all documents as required.

Following these rules enhances communication between all members of the health care team and ensures reimbursement for your facility.

Documenting completely, concisely, and accurately

Here are a few quick tips for documenting as well as you possibly can:

- Provide information that is exact and to the point.
- Use simple, precise language.
- Don't document opinions or judgments.

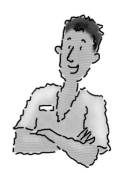

Say what?

If you don't use these tips, a rambling, vague, and ultimately meaningless documentation may occur, such as *Communication with patient's home initiated today to delineate progression of disease process and describe course of action.* That's mostly meaningless.

Instead, put your documentation tips to work, and your clear communication will occur. Here's how this information should be documented: *I contacted Andrea Sovak's daughter by phone at 1300 hours and explained that her mother's respiratory status had worsened and that she was transferred to the ICU for closer monitoring.* Documenting in this manner clearly differentiates your actions from those of the patient, the practitioner, or another staff member. (See *Tell it like it is.*)

> Don't be shy; say "I."

Don't be wishy-washy

Because we are taught that nurses don't make diagnoses, many of us qualify our observations with words like *appears* or *apparently*. However, using vague language when documenting communicates to the reader that you aren't sure what you're describing or doing. The right approach is to clearly and succinctly describe what occurred without sounding tentative.

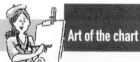

Art of the chart

Tell it like it is

In the examples below, the first is incomplete, leaving the reader wondering what really happened. The second is both complete and precise.

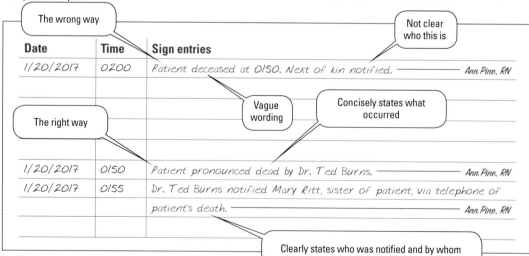

Maintaining objectivity

Knowing what to document is important, too. Record just the facts—exactly what you see, hear, and do—not your opinions or assumptions. Chart only relevant information relating to patient care and reflecting the nursing process.

Don't put words in other people's mouths

Avoid subjective statements such as *Patient's level of cooperation has deteriorated since yesterday.* Instead, use the patient's exact words to describe the facts that led you to this conclusion. You might document: *The patient stated, "I don't want to learn how to inject myself with insulin. I tried yesterday, but I'm not going to do it today."* (See *Quotations are key*.)

Art of the chart

Quotations are key

Using the patient's exact words makes your documentation accurate and objective. The notes below show how.

> Use the patient's own words as much as possible.

Date	Time	
02/10/2017	1300	Pt states she has been "voiding" drops of bloody urine every 5 to 10 minutes for the last hour. She states she feels "pressure" and a "burning pain" with voiding. Pt rates pain is a "7" on a scale of 1 to 10, in which 10 is the most severe. Dr. K. Jones's answering service notified. Dr. K. Jones will call back. ——————— Tina Clark, RN
02/10/2017	1310	Spoke with Dr. K. Jones regarding pt's symptoms. Order given for Bactrim DS, one, P.O. now and Pyridium 200 mg P.O. now. Dr. K. Jones will see pt this afternoon. ——————— Tina Clark, RN
02/10/2017	1320	Bactrim DS, one P.O. and Pyridium 200 mg P.O. given. Discussed medication uses and adverse effects; encouraged to drink plenty of fluids. I explained that Pyridium may stain clothing and turn urine orange-red. Pt, stated "I understand" and had no further questions. ——————— Tina Clark, RN
	1420	Pt states she has no pain with voiding and that "pressure is also gone." ——————— Tina Clark, RN

> Special instructions are documented precisely.

> Here's proof of patient teaching.

Secondhand data

Document only data that you collect or observe yourself or data from a reliable source, such as the patient or another nurse. When you include data reported by someone else, always cite your source. For example, you may write, *Nurse Ray found pt attempting to climb OOB. Pt was assisted to the bathroom, then back to bedside chair.*

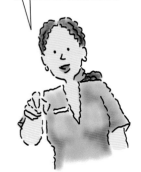

Remember to stick to the facts and leave out opinions.

Ensuring timeliness

Timely documentation includes these essentials:
* documenting as soon as possible—events sometimes get blurred or forgotten as time goes on
* documenting chronologically, noting the time of events so an accurate story can be told
* handling late entries correctly so that all necessary information is documented.

Document ASAP

Record information on the patient's medical record as soon as possible after you make an observation or provide care. Information documented immediately is more likely to be accurate and complete. If you leave your documentation until the end of the shift, you might forget important details.

One way to document on time is to enter data into the medical record at the patient's bedside. This is more easily accomplished when using an electronic health record for documentation and facilities provide beside computers. However, this system can compromise confidentiality. (See *Keeping it confidential.*)

If your facility uses computerized documentation, be sure to note if the system automatically records the events as occurring at the date

Advice from the experts

Keeping it confidential

Bedside computers are the ultimate in timely documentation, and bedside flow sheets or progress notes run a close second. However, facility policy must be followed to ensure compliance with confidentiality protocols and regulations.

One solution is to keep confidential records in a locked, fold-down desk outside the patient's room. Having a handy writing surface also makes it easier to document promptly. If your facility doesn't use bedside forms or computers, keep a worksheet or pad in your pocket for note-keeping. Jot down key phrases and times and then transcribe the information onto the medical record later.

and time that the entry is made, or if you can change the date and time to reflect when the event occurred.

Give them the time of day

Be specific about times in your documentation, especially the exact time of sudden changes in the patient's condition, significant events, and nursing actions. Don't document in blocks of time such as 0700 to 1500. This implies inattention to the patient and makes it hard to determine when specific events occurred. (See *Marking time.*)

Most facilities require nurses to chart in military time, which expresses time as 24 one-hour-long periods per day, rather than two sets of 12 one-hour periods. (See *Time marches on*, page 104.)

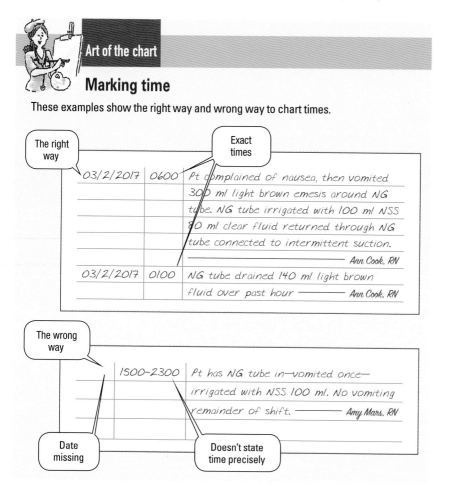

Art of the chart

Marking time

These examples show the right way and wrong way to chart times.

The right way

Exact times

03/2/2017	0600	Pt complained of nausea, then vomited 300 ml light brown emesis around NG tube. NG tube irrigated with 100 ml NSS 80 ml clear fluid returned through NG tube connected to intermittent suction.
		— Ann Cook, RN
03/2/2017	0100	NG tube drained 140 ml light brown fluid over past hour ——— Ann Cook, RN

The wrong way

| | 1500–2300 | Pt has NG tube in—vomited once— irrigated with NSS 100 ml. No vomiting remainder of shift. ——— Amy Mars, RN |

Date missing

Doesn't state time precisely

Time marches on

Many facilities use military time because it alleviates confusion over a.m. and p.m. entries. Here's how it works.

0000 hours = 12 a.m. (midnight)   1200 hours = 12 noon
0100 hours = 1 a.m.   1300 hours = 1 p.m.
0200 hours = 2 a.m.   1400 hours = 2 p.m.
0300 hours = 3 a.m.   1500 hours = 3 p.m.
0400 hours = 4 a.m.   1600 hours = 4 p.m.
0500 hours = 5 a.m.   1700 hours = 5 p.m.
0600 hours = 6 a.m.   1800 hours = 6 p.m.
0700 hours = 7 a.m.   1900 hours = 7 p.m.
0800 hours = 8 a.m.   2000 hours = 8 p.m.
0900 hours = 9 a.m.   2100 hours = 9 p.m.
1000 hours = 10 a.m.   2200 hours = 10 p.m.
1100 hours = 11 a.m.   2300 hours = 11 p.m.

Put your documentation in order

Most assessments and observations are useful only as parts of a whole picture. Isolated assessments reveal very little but, in chronologic order, they tell the patient's story over time and reveal a pattern of improvement or deterioration.

Documenting in chronologic order is easy if you jot down your observations and assessments when they occur. Too often, however, nurses document at the end of a shift and then record groups of assessments that may fail to accurately reflect variations in the patient's condition over time. (See *Correct and chronologic*, page 105.)

If you're using computerized records, know that many software programs require nurses to answer predetermined questions or fields with multiple choice answers. Although this approach will capture core data and prompt responses to key issues, it will never replace a patient-specific narrative note. If possible, combine a narrative note with the prompted documentation.

Review the documentation entries for the previous 24 to 48 hours. If the documentation is so generic that you can't identify the patient, then you'll need to incorporate narrative notes in your documentation.

Better late than never

You may occasionally need to add a late entry in certain situations, such as:
- when the chart or computer is unavailable at the time of the event
- if you forgot to document something
- if you need to add important information.

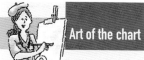

Art of the chart

Correct and chronologic

Here's an example of documentation that's done correctly in chronologic order.

Events are documented in correct time sequence.

01/14/2017	0800	Pt AAO x 3, follows commands, moves all extremities, speech clear and appropriate. Afebrile; skin warm, dry and intact; palpable pulses; no edema. Bilateral breath sounds, no shortness of breath, lungs clear, on room air. ———————————————————————— Jane Klass, RN
01/14/2017	0915	Pt complaining of sudden shortness of breath, O₂ 2 L/minute applied. Stat chest X-ray obtained, Dr. Kenneth Jones notified. ———————— Jane Klass, RN
01/14/2017	0920	Lasix 40 mg I.V. provided to pt per Dr. Kenneth Jones's order. ————————————————————————————— Jane Klass, RN
01/14/2017	0930	Shortness of breath continues, pulse oximetry 87%, O₂ increased to 50% face mask. ——————————————————— Jane Klass, RN
01/14/2017	0935	Pt transferred to ICU, report provided to Sally Brown, RN. Pt's family notified by Dr. Kenneth Jones. ————————— Jane Klass, RN

Bear in mind, however, that late entries can look suspicious if a malpractice suit occurs. Find out if your facility has a protocol for late entries. If not, add the entry on the first available line for paper documentation and label it *late entry* to indicate that it's out of sequence. Then record the date and time of the entry as well as the date and time when the entry should have been made. A computerized system may allow you to enter the information using the date and time of the event, but the software will also note the date and time of the actual entry.

Ensuring legibility

One of the main reasons to document your nursing care is to communicate patient care and condition to other members of the health care team. Whether writing a note or simply using a flow sheet, attempting to decipher a sloppy entry wastes people's time and puts the patient in jeopardy if critical information is misinterpreted, not to mention that the documentation could be misinterpreted if a legal

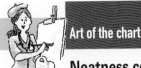

Art of the chart

Neatness counts!

Make sure your handwriting is as neat and clear as possible. Legible documentation is vital in communications among colleagues. The flow sheet below shows legible and illegible documentation.

BLOOD GLUCOSE MONITORING FLOW SHEET

Date	Time	Result	Signature	Intervention
1/5/2017	0100	106 (see progress note)	Joseph Bots, RN	N/A
1/5/2017	0700	*Pt feels nervous had meg headache*	*DErb RN*	*gave OJ Doctor in for rounds - saw pt*

The right way

The wrong way

Misspelled words and sloppy writing

This should be in the progress notes, because space here is limited.

case occurs. Use printing instead of cursive writing because it's usually easier to understand. (See *Neatness counts!*)

No pencils, please

Because it's a permanent document, the paper forms used for the clinical record should be completed in only black or blue ink, preferably black. Many paper records are scanned into a computer for storage, and using the appropriate ink makes the record more legible. Felt-tipped pens are not recommended.

Spelling counts

Notes filled with misspelled words and incorrect grammar create the same negative impression as illegible handwriting. Try hard to avoid these errors; information can be misrepresented or misconstrued if an error-filled medical record ends up in court. (See *Tips for improving spelling and grammar*, page 107.)

Tips for improving spelling and grammar

Want to look smart when you document? Here are a few pointers:
* Keep both standard and medical dictionaries in documentation areas, and refer to them as needed.
* Post a list of commonly misspelled or confusing words, especially terms and medications regularly used on the unit. Many medications have very similar names but extremely different actions.
* If your computer system includes a spelling or grammar check, use it. Understand, however, these are far from foolproof and don't replace careful proofreading.

Using abbreviations appropriately

Standards set by The Joint Commission and many state regulations stipulate that health care facilities develop a list of approved abbreviations to use during documentation. (See *Avoid these abbreviations!* page 108.) Make sure you know and use your facility's approved abbreviations. When you have doubts about a word's abbreviation, spell it out.

Using unapproved or ambiguous abbreviations can endanger a patient. For example, if you use *o.d.* for "once daily," another nurse might think you mean "oculus dexter" (right eye) and instill medication into the patient's eye instead of giving it orally. (See *Acceptable vs. unacceptable abbreviations,* page 110.)

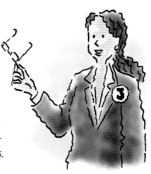

Correcting errors properly

When you make a mistake in the patient's medical record, correct it immediately by drawing a single line through the entry and writing *error* or *mistaken entry* above or beside it, along with the date and time. Then sign your name or initials. Never erase a mistake, cover it with correction fluid, or completely cross it out because this looks as if you're trying to hide something. Also, writing *oops* or *sorry* or drawing a happy or sad face anywhere on a document is unprofessional and inappropriate. (See *Correct correctly!* page 110.)

Changing a record in any way is illegal and constitutes tampering. If the patient's medical record ends up in court, the plaintiff's lawyer will be looking for red flags that cast doubt on the medical record's accuracy. (See *Altered records,* page 111.) So heed the following list of five "don'ts":
1. Don't add information at a later date without indicating that you did so by inserting the date and time of the entry and writing "late entry."

An important documentation rule: Never erase a mistake.

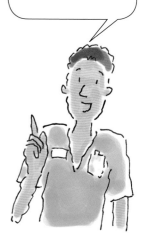

Avoid these abbreviations!

The Joint Commission requires every health care facility to develop a list of approved abbreviations for staff use. Certain abbreviations should be avoided because they're easily misunderstood, especially when handwritten. The Joint Commission has identified a minimum list of dangerous abbreviations, acronyms, and symbols. Additionally, the Institute for Safe Medication Practices has a more extensive list which is available on their web site www.ismp.org. Computerized provider order entry has safety steps built in because a computerized system is built to not allow the practitioner to choose an unacceptable abbreviation. Do-Not-Use lists usually include the following items.

Abbreviation	Intended meaning	Misinterpretation	Correction
U or u	unit	Frequently misinterpreted as a "0" or a "4," or "cc" causing a tenfold or greater overdose	Write "unit."
IU	international unit	Frequently misinterpreted as intravenous (I.V.) or 10	Write "International Unit."
q.d., qd, QD, Q.D. q.o.d., qod, QOD, Q.O.D.	every day every other day	Mistaken for each other. The period after the "q" has sometimes been misinterpreted as "i," the "o" can be mistaken for "i," and the drug has been given q.i.d. rather than daily.	Write "daily" or "every other day."
Trailing zero (X.0 mg) Lack of leading zero (.X mg)	10 mg, 0.1 mg	Frequently misinterpreted dosage as the decimal point is missed	Never write a zero by itself after a decimal point (10.0 mg should be 10 mg) and always use a zero before a decimal point if no other number is present, such as 0.1 mg.
MS, MSO₄, MgSO₄	morphine sulfate magnesium sulfate	Confused with each other	Write "morphine sulfate" or "magnesium sulfate."

In addition to the minimum required list, the following items should also be considered when expanding the Do-Not-Use list.

ʒ	fluid dram	Misinterpreted as "3"	Use the metric equivalents.
♍	minim	Misinterpreted as "ml"	Use the metric equivalents.
MTX	methotrexate	Misinterpreted as mustargen (mechlorethamine hydrochloride)	Write "methotrexate."
CPZ	Compazine (prochlorperazine)	Misinterpreted as chlorpromazine	Write "Compazine."
HCl	hydrochloric acid	Misinterpreted as potassium chloride ("H" is misinterpreted as "K")	Write "hydrochloric acid."

Avoid these abbreviations! *(continued)*

Abbreviation	Intended meaning	Misinterpretation	Correction
HCTZ	hydrochlorothiazide	Misinterpreted as hydrocortisone (HCT)	Write "hydrochlorothiazide."
TNK	TNKase	Misinterpreted as "TPN"	Write "TNKase."
au	*auris uterque* (each ear)	Frequently misinterpreted as "OU" (*oculus uterque*—each eye)	Write "each ear."
μg	microgram	Frequently misinterpreted as "mg"	Use "mcg."
cc	cubic centimeter	Frequently misinterpreted as U (units)	Write "ml" for milliliters.
A.S., A.D., and AU	Latin abbreviations for left ear, right ear, and both ears, respectively	Frequently misinterpreted as O.S., O.D., and OU	Write "left ear," "right ear," or "both ears."
OD	once daily	Frequently misinterpreted as "O.D." (*oculus dexter*—right eye)	Write "once daily."
OJ	orange juice	Frequently misinterpreted as "O.D." (*oculus dexter*—right eye) or "O.S." (*oculus sinister*—left eye). Medications that were meant to be diluted in orange juice and given orally have been given in a patient's right or left eye.	Write "orange juice."
Per os	orally	The "os" is frequently misinterpreted as "O.S." (*oculus sinister*—left eye).	Use "PO," "by mouth," or "orally."
qn.	nightly or at bedtime	Frequently misinterpreted as "q.h." (every hour)	Write out "nightly" or "at bedtime."
S.C., subq, SQ	subcutaneous	Mistaken as SL for sublingual or "5 every"	Use "subcut," or write out "subcutaneous."
D/C	discharge or discontinue	Frequently misinterpreted as each other	Write "discharge" or "discontinue."
h.s.	half-strength or at bedtime	Frequently misinterpreted as each other	Write out "half-strength" or "at bedtime."
T.I.W.	three times per week	Frequently misinterpreted as three times per day or twice weekly	Write "three times per week."

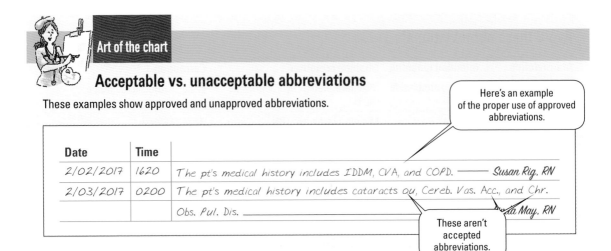

Art of the chart

Acceptable vs. unacceptable abbreviations

These examples show approved and unapproved abbreviations.

Here's an example of the proper use of approved abbreviations.

Date	Time	
2/02/2017	1620	The pt's medical history includes IDDM, CVA, and COPD. ——— Susan Rig, RN
2/03/2017	0200	The pt's medical history includes cataracts ou, Cereb. Vas. Acc., and Chr.
		Obs. Pul. Dis. ——————————————— ...a May, RN

These aren't accepted abbreviations.

2. Don't date the entry so that it appears to have been written at an earlier time.
3. Don't add inaccurate or false information.
4. Don't omit information.
5. Don't destroy records.

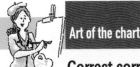

Art of the chart

Correct correctly!

When you make a mistake on the clinical record, correct it by drawing a single line through the entry and writing *error* or the words *mistaken entry* above or beside it (don't use an abbreviation like *m.e.*, which could be someone's initials). Follow this with your initials and the date. If appropriate, briefly explain why the correction was necessary.

Make sure that the mistaken entry is still legible to indicate that you're only trying to correct a mistake, not cover something up.

The right way to correct an error

Date	Time	Sign entries
02/10/2017	0900	error N.C. 02/10/2017 ~~Pt. states he is dizzy when changing from sitting to standing position~~
		——————————————————— Nancy Cobb, RN

The wrong, illegal way

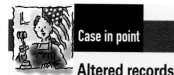

Case in point

Altered records

Cagnolatti v. Hightower (1996) is an example of the consequences of altering records. In this case, a 72-year-old female patient was admitted to the hospital after having a stroke. The night before discharge, the nurse assisted the practitioner in administering intravenous (I.V.) edrophonium (Tensilon). Shortly after the drug's administration, the patient developed adverse reactions. The drug was discontinued. Most of the patient's symptoms disappeared within 15 minutes of stopping the drug. However, about 30 minutes after the drug was stopped, the patient went into cardiac arrest. The patient was resuscitated but remained comatose and died about 2 months later.

Record review
The patient's pulse after drug administration was documented as 88 beats/minute, but the nurse testified that this heart rate was likely obtained before the drug was given. Documentation also showed that the patient's heart rate was 88 beats/minute 15 minutes after drug administration. However, a handwriting expert testified that the second heart rate was originally entered as 58 beats/minute and had been altered to appear as 88 beats/minute. In addition, there was no documentation that a nursing assessment was performed during the 30-minute period after the drug was stopped.

The verdict
Any heart rate less than 60 beats/minute is considered bradycardic and requires intervention, especially after edrophonium administration. The heart rate should have been brought to the attention of the treating practitioner. Furthermore, the nurse should have monitored the patient more closely and documented the results of the assessment.

If your facility uses computerized records, follow the protocols for the correction of entries made in the chart. Once notes are entered into the computer, they become the permanent record and shouldn't be deleted or edited at a later time without an explanation that's documented, signed, and dated.

Signing documents

Sign each entry you make in the progress notes with your first name or initial, last name, and professional licensure, such as registered nurse (RN) or licensed practical nurse (LPN). Your employer may also require that you include your job title. If you find the last entry unsigned, immediately contact the nurse who made the entry and ask the nurse to sign the entry. If you can't locate the nurse, simply write and sign your progress notes. The difference in documentation times

Art of the chart

Documentation do's and don'ts

The samples below illustrate some important rules about documentation.

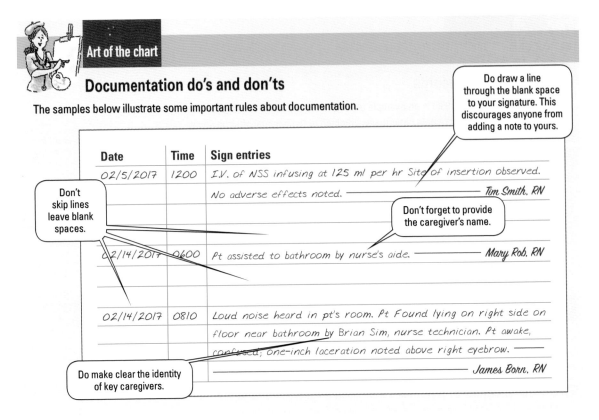

Do draw a line through the blank space to your signature. This discourages anyone from adding a note to yours.

Don't skip lines leave blank spaces.

Don't forget to provide the caregiver's name.

Do make clear the identity of key caregivers.

Date	Time	Sign entries
02/5/2017	1200	I.V. of NSS infusing at 125 ml per hr Site of insertion observed.
		No adverse effects noted. ———————— Tim Smith, RN
02/14/2017	0600	Pt assisted to bathroom by nurse's aide. ———————— Mary Rob, RN
02/14/2017	0810	Loud noise heard in pt's room. Pt found lying on right side on floor near bathroom by Brian Sim, nurse technician. Pt awake, confused; one-inch laceration noted above right eyebrow. ———
		———————————————— James Born, RN

and handwriting should make it clear who the author was. (See *Documentation do's and don'ts*.)

To be continued . . .

When documentation continues from one page to the next, sign the bottom of the first page. At the top of the next page, write the date, the time, and *continued from previous page*. Make sure that each page is stamped or labeled with the patient's identifying information.

Never leave blank spaces on forms. Doing so could imply that you failed to give complete care or to assess the patient completely. If information listed on a form doesn't apply to your patient, write *N/A* (not applicable) in the space. If your documentation doesn't fill the designated space, draw a line through the empty space until you reach your signature.

What you didn't see can hurt you

If you need to document the actions of nursing assistants or technicians, write the caregiver's full name—not just initials. Many nurses worry about countersigning care that they didn't actually see performed. If this is the case, you may refer to your facility's policy, contact your state board of nursing, or discuss the issue with your nurse-manager. Remember, your signature makes you responsible for everything in the notes.

If your facility uses electronic health records, know that most software programs establish an electronic signature based on your personal user password. It's extremely important to guard your password and not share it with others. This is your legal signature! Always be sure to log off when leaving the computer station. Don't allow anyone else to use the computer with your password logged in. Any entries another person makes while you are logged in will be stamped with your electronic signature. Some electronic health systems also create a system to cosign another's documentation, such as a certified nurse assistant or nursing student. Be aware that this cosignature confirms your agreement with the information documented.

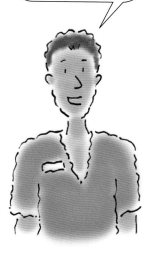

Write out the full names of nursing assistants or technicians when documenting their actions.

Practitioner's orders

Almost every treatment you give a patient requires a practitioner's or a licensed independent practitioner's order, so accurate documentation of these orders is critical. Orders fall into four categories:

1. written or electronic orders
2. preprinted orders
3. verbal orders
4. telephone orders.

Written or electronic orders

No matter who transcribes an order—an RN, an LPN, or a unit secretary—a second person must double-check the transcription for accuracy. Electronic orders may need verification by an RN before they are sent to respective departments, such as radiology or laboratory. An effective method to check written orders is the "chart check"—rechecking orders from the previous shift. This is often part of the hand-off process that occurs between shifts.

Additionally, checking for transcription errors at least once every 24 hours is also a good idea. These checks are usually done on the night shift. Once completed, a line is placed across the order sheet to indicate that all orders above the line have been checked. "24-hour chart check" may be written and then the sheet is signed and dated to document when the check was done and by whom. Electronic health systems may have its own system for checking orders. Follow the procedure based on the specific electronic health system used in your facility.

Heading off mistakes

When checking a patient's order sheet, make sure that the orders were written for the right patient. An order sheet might be stamped with one patient's identification plate and then inadvertently placed in another patient's chart. Double-checking averts potential mistakes.

If an order is unclear or illegible, call the practitioner who wrote the order for clarification. Don't ask other people for their interpretation; they'll only be guessing, too. If a practitioner is notorious for poor handwriting, ask the practitioner to review all written orders with you or the charge nurse before leaving the unit.

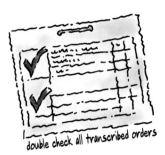

double check all transcribed orders

If you use electronic documentation, be aware that some programs allow you to select more than one patient at a time. Be sure to double-check the patient's name on the computer screen before entering orders given by a practitioner.

Some facilities that use an electronic system require the practitioners to enter all of their orders into the system under a specific physician's order entry program. This system greatly reduces errors because it eliminates transcription. However, it's still important to check for accuracy and make sure orders are entered for the right patient.

Preprinted orders

Many health care facilities use preprinted order forms for specific procedures, such as cardiac catheterization or for admission to certain units such as the coronary care unit. As with other standardized documents, blank spaces are used for information that must be individualized according to the patient's needs.

If your facility uses these forms, don't assume that they're flawless just because they're preprinted. You may still need to clarify an order by discussing it with the practitioner who gave it. (See *Preprinted orders*, page 115.)

Verbal orders

Verbal orders are easy to misinterpret and are discouraged by certifying agencies, such as The Joint Commission. Errors in understanding or documenting such orders can cause errors in patient care and liability problems for you and your facility. Try to take verbal orders only in an emergency when the practitioner can't immediately attend to the patient. As a rule, do-not-resuscitate and no-code orders should *not* be taken verbally.

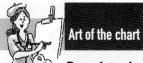

Art of the chart

Preprinted orders

The following is an example of a preprinted form for documenting practitioner's orders. This form specifies the treatment for a patient who's about to undergo cardiac catheterization.

PHYSICIAN ORDERS

Allergies: *None known*

Date/Time	PRECARDIAC CATHETERIZATION ORDERS:
2/1/2017 0130	1. NPO after *midnight* except for sips of water with medications.
	2. Shave and prep right and left groin areas.
	3. Premedications:
	Benadryl _25_ mg } P.O. on call to Cath lab
	Xanax _0.5_ mg
	4. Have ECG, PT, PTT, creatinine, Hgb, Hct, and platelet count on chart prior to sending
	the patient to the Cath lab.
	5. Have patient void before leaving for the Cath lab.
2/1/2017 0130	*John Smith, MD* ————————
2/1/2017 0200	*noted/Mona Jones, RN* ————————

> Blanks are left for information that should be individualized according to the patient's needs.

From words to paper

Carefully follow your facility's policy for documenting verbal orders, using a special form if one exists. Here's the usual procedure:

- Record the order verbatim on the physician's order sheet or enter it into a computer. Note the date and time.
- On the first line, write "verbal order." Then write the practitioner's name and your name as the nurse who received the order. When using a computer, it will usually require documentation of what type of order is being logged. Choose "verbal order."
- *Read the order back to the practitioner for confirmation that you understood the order correctly, and receive verification from the person who gave the order. (This step is called "The Joint Commission read back requirement" and applies to all verbal and telephone orders.)*

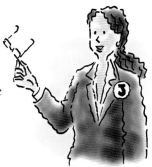

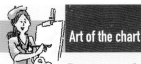

Documenting verbal orders

This form shows the correct way to document verbal orders. Make sure that the practitioner countersigns the order within the designated time frame per facility policy.

PHYSICIAN ORDERS	
Date/Time	**Sign entries**
1/16/2017 1500	Lasix 40mg IV now and daily starting in am.
	Verbal order from Dr. J. Marks with readback verification ————
	———————————————————————— Mary Jones, RN

- Sign your name.
- Draw lines through any space between the order and your verification of the order.
- When taking a medication order as a verbal order, include the type of drug, the dosage, the route, the timing of administration (such as "stat," twice a day [b.i.d.], etc.), and any other pertinent information. (See *Documenting verbal orders*.)
- Make sure the practitioner countersigns the order within the time limits set by your facility. Without a countersignature, you may be held liable for practicing medicine without a license.

Telephone orders

Ideally, you should accept only written or electronic orders from a practitioner. However, telephone orders are permissible when:
- the patient needs immediate treatment and the practitioner isn't available to write or enter an order
- you're providing care to the patient at home (If so, the orders must be signed by the practitioner according to state nursing practice regulations. Under Medicare guidelines, verbal orders must be signed within 30 days. Other agencies impose their own, stricter rules. Failure to obtain a signed order could jeopardize reimbursement.)

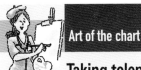

Art of the chart

Taking telephone orders

This form shows the correct way to document telephone orders. Make sure that the practitioner countersigns the order.

PHYSICIAN ORDERS	
Date/Time	**Sign entries**
2/4/2017 0900	Morphine sulfate 2 mg I.V. now for pain.
	Telephone order from Dr. M. Barthlomew with readback verification
	———————————————————— *Cathy Phillips, RN*

- new information (laboratory data, for example) has become available, and the telephone order will enable you to expedite care. (See *Taking telephone orders*.)

From phone to paper

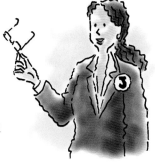

Telephone orders should be given directly to you; they should never go through a third party. Carefully follow your facility's policy for documenting these orders. Usually, you'll follow this procedure:

- Record the order verbatim on the physician's order sheet or enter it into a computer. First, note the date and time. On the next line, write "telephone order." (Don't use *P.O.* for phone order—it could be mistaken for "by mouth.") Then write the practitioner's name, and sign your name.
- *Read the order back to the practitioner for confirmation that you understood the order correctly, and receive verification from the person who gave the order. (This step is called "The Joint Commission read back requirement" and applies to all verbal and telephone orders. The read back requirement also applies to critical test results reported verbally or by telephone.)*
- If you're having trouble understanding the practitioner, ask another nurse to listen in as the practitioner gives you the order. Then have the nurse read it back and sign the order, too.
- Draw lines through any blank spaces in the order.
- Make sure that the practitioner countersigns the order within the time limits set by your facility. Without the signature, you may be held liable for practicing medicine without a license.

- To save time and avoid errors (and if permitted by your facility's confidentiality policy), ask the practitioner to fax you a copy of the order. Make sure that you wait at the fax machine for the transmission to protect the patient's right to confidentiality.

Questioning practitioner's orders

Although the unit secretary may transcribe orders, you're ultimately responsible for the transcription's accuracy.

Chart authority

Only you have the authority and the knowledge to question the validity of orders and to spot errors. This is why a chart check is so important.

Stop, question, and document

What if an order seems vague or incorrect? Refuse to carry it out until you talk to the practitioner to clarify the order. (See *When in doubt, check it out* and *Failure to question*.)

Your facility should have a written procedure for clarifying orders. If it doesn't, take these steps:

- Contact the prescribing practitioner for clarification.
- Document the date and time that you made this contact.
- Document any changes to the order and whether you carried out the order.
- If you refuse to carry out an order, document your refusal, including the reasons why you refused and your communications with the practitioner. Inform your immediate supervisor.
- Ask your nursing administrator for a step-by-step policy to follow so you'll know what to do if the situation recurs.

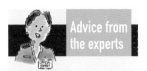

When in doubt, check it out

An order may be correct when issued but incorrect later because of changes in the patient's status. When this occurs, delay the treatment until you have contacted the practitioner and clarified the situation.

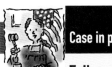

Case in point

Failure to question

In *Poor Sisters of Saint Francis Seraph of the Perpetual Adoration, et al. v. Catron (1982)*, a hospital was sued for negligence because a nurse failed to question a practitioner's order regarding an endotracheal tube.

The practitioner ordered that the tube be left in place for 5 days instead of the standard 2 to 3 days. The nurse knew that 5 days was exceptionally long but, instead of clarifying the practitioner's order, the order was carried out. As a result, the patient's larynx was irreparably damaged, and the court ruled the hospital negligent.

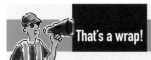

That's a wrap!

Expert documentation review

Seven fundamental rules

- Document completely, concisely, and accurately.
- Avoid using opinions; stick to the facts.
- Document in a timely manner, making sure the information is in chronologic order and noting exact times.
- Make sure your documentation is legible. (Use printing instead of cursive, and use black or blue ink.)
- Use only accepted abbreviations.
- Follow protocols for correcting documentation errors and adding late entries.
- Sign your notes with your first name or initial, last name, and licensure.

Practitioner's orders

- *Written or electronic*—double-check all orders and clarify them, if necessary.
- *Preprinted*—orders must be individualized according to the patient's needs; don't assume they're flawless; you may still need to clarify an order.
- *Verbal*—take verbal orders only in an emergency, and make sure the practitioner countersigns within the time limits set by your facility.
- *Telephone*—take telephone orders only under certain circumstances, and make sure to take the order yourself.

Suggested references

Institute of Safe Medication Practices. "ISMP's List of Error-Prone Abbreviations, Symbols, and Dose Designations," 2015. Available: http://www.ismp.org/Tools/errorproneabbreviations.pdf.

Nursing Care Quality Assurance Commission. "Advisory Opinion: Standing Orders and Verbal Orders," 2014. Available: https://www.doh.wa.gov/Portals/1/Documents/6000/StandingAndVerbalOrders.pdf.

The Joint Commission. "Facts About the Official 'Do Not Use' List of Abbreviations," 2017. Available: https://www.jointcommission.org/facts_about_do_not_use_list/.

The Joint Commission. "What Did the Doctor Say?: Improving Health Literacy to Protect Patient Safety," 2007. Available: https://www.jointcommission.org/what_did_the_doctor_say/.

Chapter 6

Avoiding legal pitfalls

Just the facts

In this chapter, you'll learn:

◆ the legal significance of the medical record

◆ defensive documentation

◆ the relationship between documentation and risk management

◆ eight documentation pitfalls and how to handle them.

A look at legal pitfalls in documentation

As your professional responsibility grows, so does your legal accountability. Timely, accurate, objective, and complete documentation proves that you're providing quality care and meeting professional and legal standards. Good documentation is your best defense and will protect you in the future if you're named in a malpractice lawsuit. Remember, if there is no documentation, there is no evidence to support the care you provided to the patient. (See *What sways the jury?* page 121.)

The aim is communication

According to the American Nurses Association (ANA) Principles for Nursing Documentation, clear, accurate, and accessible documentation is an essential element of safe, quality, evidence-based nursing practice. Additionally, the medical record must be specific and describes who did, what, when, and how. Inaccurate, unclear, incomplete, or missing documentation can expose you to potential litigation and the care you provided to be questioned as medical records are scrutinized by health care experts and presented in court case trials. Think of the medical record as a communication tool which proves and confirms that care was provided. Document accordingly, focus on the facts, be objective, and document chronologically.

What sways the jury?

The outcome of every malpractice case that goes to trial boils down to one question: Who will the jury believe? The answer depends on the credibility of the evidence. Jurors usually view the medical record as the best evidence of what really happened. It's commonly the hinge on which the verdict swings.

A general overview

In a nutshell, here's what happens in court if a lawsuit is brought against you: The plaintiff's (patient's) lawyer presents evidence showing that the patient was harmed and that the nurse "caused" the harm because the care provided (or not provided and should have been) by the defendant (in this case, the nurse) failed to meet accepted standards of care. The defendant's (nurse's) lawyer presents evidence showing that you, the client, provided a standard of care that would be used by other nurses given the same or similar circumstances and therefore met the standard of care.

The medical record provides the best evidence of what happened with the patient and is used to evaluate the quality of care the patient received, including if the standard of care was met. Incomplete and inaccurate documentation is the primary issue in malpractice cases and is the plaintiff's best evidence when trying to show or prove that the standard of care was not met. The jury will almost certainly rule in favor of the patient if documentation in the medical record does not support that the standard of care was met and that quality of care was not optimal. Don't believe the myth that all cases settle out of court. Most do, but you don't want to be the exception.

Remember, charts are communication tools first and foremost.

Legal standards

Standards of care are governed by:
- state nurse practice acts (NPAs)
- accreditation organizations/federal regulations
- ANA
- your facility's policies and procedures.

Nurse practice acts

NPAs are state laws that govern the profession of nursing. Each state's NPA is passed by the state's legislature and establishes a Board of Nursing (BON) that has the authority to develop additional administrative rules and regulations to help clarify or to make the NPA more specific. The BON is responsible for the regulation of nursing and enforcement of the law. Remember, ignorance of the law is never an excuse for not practicing within the limits of the law. It's your responsibility to become familiar with your state's NPA through your state BON.

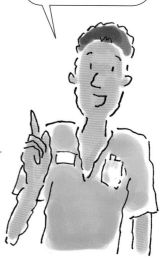

In a confused state? Read on . . .

The range of a nurse's legal responsibilities and capabilities may vary from state to state—perhaps only to a small degree in certain cases. However, if licensed in more than one state, you must take care to become knowledgeable about specific laws and follow them precisely including the legal scope of practice in the state you're practicing. You'll be held liable if you're found practicing outside of your designated scope of practice as defined by state law.

Accreditation organizations/federal regulations

Accrediting organizations for hospitals, such as The Joint Commission (TJC), Healthcare Facilities Accreditation Program (HFAP), and Det Norske Veritas (DNV) Healthcare Inc. grants recognition for demonstrated ability to meet preestablished criteria for established standards, some of which further define nursing process and practice.

Accrediting organizations may incorporate federal regulations such as Conditions of Participation for Hospital, which outline the criteria to meet for hospitals to participate in Medicare and Medicaid programs.

Whatever accrediting organization your facility uses, become familiar with those standards that relate to nursing process and practice, including the Conditions of Participation for Hospital if applicable, so that your practice is compliant with those standards.

ANA credentialing

What you write in a medical record shouldn't be dictated by the courts; it should be guided by the nursing profession's own standards. Documentation that meets these high-quality standards describes the patient's status, medical treatment, and nursing care, which is reflective of the nursing process. The ANA sets documentation standards for most nursing specialties. It states that documentation must be:

- clear, concise, and complete
- timely, in order (sequential), and contemporaneous
- accessible and retrievable on a permanent basis
- accurate, relevant, and consistent
- recorded in a way that allows it to be audited
- legible and readable—this applies to both written documents and an electronic health record (EHR) entries.

The more things change, the more they stay the same

Although documentation goals haven't changed much over the years, documentation methods have. Nurses now use standardized flow sheets, graphic records, and checklists in place of long narrative notes. Many or all of these are now embedded into EHR systems. In malpractice cases, the method of documentation used isn't important, as long as it's used consistently and provides comprehensive, factual information that's relevant to the patient's care so that it can be used to provide evidence of the care provided, which can help in your defense.

Malpractice litigation

When documenting, your main goal is to convey and communicate information. However, keep the legal implications in the back of your mind. If the care you provide and your documentation are both top-notch, the records may be used to refute a plaintiff's accusation of nursing malpractice.

A malpractice verdict depends on three factors which the plaintiff's lawyer must prove:
1. breach of duty—which refers to your duty to provide the standard of care. This may be an act of commission or omission (something you *did* or something you *should have* done).
2. damage—referring to the patient being harmed
3. causation—the breach of duty caused harm.

Every relationship brings with it responsibility

The courts have ruled that it's your duty to provide an appropriate standard of care once a nurse–patient relationship is established—even if the relationship takes place over the phone. Breach of duty means that your care didn't meet the standards of care.

Proving that a nurse was guilty of breach of duty is difficult because the nurse's duties overlap with those of other health care providers. The court will ask, "How would a reasonable, prudent nurse with comparable training and experience have acted in the same or a similar circumstance?"

Once the plaintiff establishes a breach of duty, it must then proven that the breach caused the patient's injury (damage and causation).

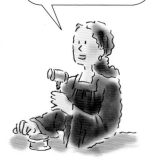

When you establish a relationship with a patient, you take on a legal responsibility.

Facility policies and procedures

How you document is also defined by the policies and procedures at your specific facility, such as facility-wide policies and procedures and/or specific nursing or unit policies and procedures. Straying from these could suggest that you failed to meet the facility's defined standards of care. Additionally, because most facilities now have EHRs and documentation is electronic, make sure you also become familiar with those policies or procedures related to "downtime" processes when the EHR is unavailable.

Although the courts have yet to decide whether these policies actually establish a legal standard of care, there are legal standards in place. In each nursing malpractice case, the courts compare a nurse's actions with regularly updated, national minimum standards established by professional organizations and accrediting bodies such as TJC.

The ties that bind

Although physicians get sued more than nurses, that trend has shifted to include other members of the health care team, including nurses. Therefore, you are accountable for the care that you provide to your patients and could be named in a lawsuit. From 1992 to 2014, the rate of paid medical malpractice claims in the United States has declined significantly, dropping about 56%. However, the average payout rose about 23%. Some states have passed legislation for medical malpractice claims, otherwise known as "tort reform." These types of laws "limit" or "cap" damage claims. Find out about and become familiar with your state's medical malpractice "tort reform" laws if applicable.

Developing a good relationship with your patients can help reduce the risk of being sued. The patient's perception of you is very important and can be a factor in filing a lawsuit. Being a good communicator and being perceived as friendly, warm, and helpful all contribute to developing a good relationship and a positive perception by the patient.

Establishing a strong nurse–patient relationship may help reduce legal risks.

Documenting defensively

In the world of nursing and malpractice, a defensive attitude has become necessary—that is, document factually but defensively as well. This involves knowing:
1. how to chart
2. what to chart
3. when to chart
4. who should chart.

How to chart

A skilled nurse charts, keeping the possibility of litigation in mind and knows how, what, and when to chart.

Rule #1: Stick to the facts

Record only what you see, hear, smell, feel, measure, and count—not what you suppose, infer, speculate, conclude, or assume. Remain objective and state the facts. For example, if a patient pulled out the intravenous (I.V.) line but you didn't witness it, write *Found pt, arm board, and bed linens covered with blood. I.V. line and venipuncture device were untaped and hanging free*. If the patient admits to pulling out the I.V. line, record that; however, do not make that assumption.

Don't chart your opinions and avoid bias. State the facts, not value judgments. If the chart is used as evidence in court, the plaintiff's lawyer might attack your credibility and the medical record's reliability.

Rule #2: Avoid labeling

Objectively describe the patient's behavior instead of subjectively labeling it or coming to your own conclusion. For example, write

Pt found pacing back and forth in the room, muttering phrases such as, "I'll take care of him my way" while punching one hand into the other. Avoid using expressions such as *appears spaced out, flying high, exhibiting bizarre behavior,* or *using obscenities,* which can mean different things to different people. Ask yourself, "Could I define these terms in court?" Objectivity in documentation will increase your credibility with the jury.

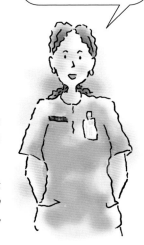

Remember, facts speak for themselves. Never chart your subjective opinions or conclusions.

Rule #3: Be specific

Your documentation goal is to present the facts clearly, concisely, and as accurately as possible. Be sure to make clear who gave the care. To do so, use only standardized, facility-approved abbreviations and express your observations in quantifiable terms whenever possible. (See *Specifics are terrific!*)

Also, avoid catch-all phrases such as *Pt comfortable, ate well, appears confused and medicated for pain* to name a few. Instead, be more specific and describe how you know this.

For example, writing *output adequate* isn't as helpful as writing *output 1,200 ml.* And *Pt appears to be in pain* is vague compared with *Pt requested pain medication after complaining of lower back pain radiating to the ⓇR leg, rated 7 out of 10 on the visual analogue scale.* Another example, instead of *ate well,* state *Pt ate 100% of the regular diet breakfast.*

Rule #4: Use neutral language

Don't use inappropriate comments or language in your notes. Do not express strong opinions or feelings. This is unprofessional and can cause legal problems.

Art of the chart

Specifics are terrific!

The note below is clear and concise because it uses approved abbreviations and specific measurements.

5/16/2017	1000	Pt c/o pain at Ⓛ antecubital I.V. site. Pain rated 3 out of 10 on scale of
		0 to 10. Redness noted 2 cm wide around I.V. insertion site with quarter-
		sized area of edema above the site. I.V. removed, site cleaned with
		chlorhexidine and sterile dressing applied. Warm compresses applied to site.
		Pt refuses pain medication. ———————————— M.Doherty RN
5/16/2017	1030	I.V. site with less redness. Pt now rates pain 0 out of 10 on scale of
		0 to 10.

In one case, an elderly patient developed pressure injuries and the family complained that the patient wasn't receiving adequate care. The patient later died, probably of natural causes. Because family members were dissatisfied with the patient's care, they sued. The insurance company questioned the abbreviation *PBBB* in the chart, which the practitioner had written under prognosis. After learning that this stood for "pine box by bedside," the family was awarded a significant sum.

Rule #5: Eliminate bias

Don't use language that suggests a negative attitude toward the patient. Examples include *obstinate, drunk, obnoxious, bizarre,* or *abusive.* The same goes for what you say out loud and then document. Disparaging remarks, accusations, arguments, or name calling could lead to a defamation of character or libel suit. In court, the plaintiff's lawyer might say, "This nurse called my client 'rude, difficult, and uncooperative.' The nurse documented it in the medical record. No wonder the nurse didn't take good care of the patient—the nurse didn't like him." Remember, the patient has a legal right to see the medical record. If the patient spots a derogatory reference, feelings may range from being hurt to feeling anger and the likelihood of suing increases.

If a patient is difficult or uncooperative, document the behavior objectively and let the jurors draw their own conclusions. (See *Polite and to the point.*)

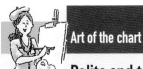

Art of the chart

Polite and to the point

The note below describes a difficult situation dispassionately while still getting the point across.

3/17/2017	1300	Patient refused the daily abdominal dressing change, stating, "This doesn't need to be done every day. It doesn't hurt and I don't want you to touch it. Leave me alone." Provided teaching regarding the importance of monitoring and cleaning the incision and offered an analgesic to be given 20 min before dressing would be changed. Pt became agitated and still refused. ——————————————— Mary Marley, RN
3/17/2017	1330	Dr. B. Humbert notified of patient's refusal of dressing change and agitated state. No new orders given. ——————— Mary Marley, RN

Rule #6: Keep the record intact

Be sure to keep the patient's chart complete. Let's say that you spill coffee on a page and blur several entries. Don't discard the original! Keep it on the chart. Discarding parts of the medical record, even for innocent reasons, raises doubt in a lawyer's mind. (See *Missing records*.)

Rule #7: Know your EHR

Be sure to take advantage of any and all opportunities on how to properly document in your facility's EHR. Also, be aware of what resources are available to you in the event you have any questions or need support. Always be sure to protect all of your passwords that allow you access to the EHR.

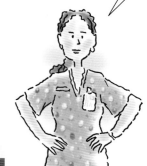

Always keep the original pages in a patient's chart.

Case in point

Missing records

The case of *Keene v. Brigham and Women's Hospital* (2003) shows how missing records can raise doubt about whether proper care was given to a patient. In this situation, a neonate developed respiratory distress and cyanosis within hours of birth. He was transferred to the neonatal intensive care unit. Blood tests, including a complete blood count and a blood culture, were performed. The patient was then transferred back to the regular nursery for "routine care" with instructions for staff to watch for signs and symptoms of sepsis and to withhold antibiotic therapy pending the results of the complete blood count. About 20 hours after the transfer, the neonate went into septic shock and started having seizures. Antibiotics were given at this time.

Record skips

Subsequent testing revealed that the neonate had neonatal sepsis and meningitis and tested positive for group B beta-hemolytic streptococci. However, no one could determine whether anyone was notified about the patient's condition or if appropriate actions were taken because about 18 hours worth of hospital records relating to the patient couldn't be found.

The verdict

The court held that a party who has negligently or intentionally lost or destroyed evidence known to be relevant for an upcoming legal proceeding should be held accountable for any unfair prejudice that results. Therefore, the court inferred that without evidence to the contrary, the missing records would have likely contained proof that the antibiotics should have been administered sooner and that the defendant's failure to do so caused the neonate's injuries.

What to document

Caring for patients seems more important than documenting every detail, doesn't it? However, legally speaking, an incomplete chart reflects incomplete nursing care. Neglecting to record every detail is such a serious and common documentation error that malpractice lawyers have coined the expression "Not charted, not done."

This doesn't mean that you have to document everything. Some information, such as staffing shortages and staff conflicts, is definitely off limits. (See *Documentation don'ts*, page 129.)

Rule #1: Document significant situations or unusual events

Learn to recognize legally dangerous situations. Be sure to document details of an unusual event, specific interventions provided to the patient and the patient's response, any patient statements, who you notified, including what you told them, and if you received any orders or changes to the plan of care. Assess each critical or out-of-the-ordinary situation, and decide whether your actions might be questioned in court. If they could be, document them as clear and concise as you can so that others who review the record will know exactly what happened and what you did in response. (See *Understanding negligence*, page 130, and *Out of the ordinary*, page 130.)

Rule #2: Document complete assessment data

Failing to perform and document a complete physical assessment is a key factor in many malpractice suits. During your initial assessment, focus on the patient's reason for seeking care and then follow up on all other problems mentioned. Be sure to chart everything you *do* as well as *why*. (See *The trouble with charting by exception*, page 131.)

After completing the initial assessment, write a well-constructed care plan. Doing so gives you a clear approach to the patient's problems and helps defend your care if you're sued.

Phrase each problem statement clearly, and modify them as you gather new assessment data. State the care plan for solving each problem and then identify the actions or interventions you intend to take. Don't forget to document the actual interventions you implement as well as the patient's response to the interventions.

Rule #3: Document discharge instructions

Because of insurance constraints, facilities are now discharging patients earlier than they once did. This change means that patients and family members are changing dressings, assessing wounds, and tackling other tasks that nurses have traditionally performed. Patient and family teaching is your responsibility. If a patient receives inadequate or incorrect instructions and an injury results, you could be held

Family teaching is part of your professional responsibility. Be sure to document all patient/family teaching and the patient's/family's level of understanding or if additional teaching is needed. Also document if you provide the patient/family any written materials.

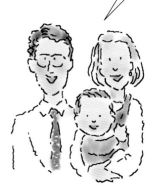

Advice from the experts

Documentation don'ts

Negative language and inappropriate information don't belong in a medical record and can return to haunt you in a lawsuit. The documentation mistakes below are legal land mines. Avoid them.

1. Don't record staffing problems
Although staff shortages may affect patient care or contribute to an incident, you shouldn't mention this in a patient's medical record because it can be used as legal ammunition against you if the medical record lands in court. Instead, write a confidential memo to your nurse-manager, and review your facility's policy and procedure manuals to see how you're expected to handle this situation.

2. Don't record staff conflicts
Don't document:
• disputes with other nurses (including criticisms of their care)
• questions about a practitioner's treatment
• a colleague's rude or abusive behavior.
   Personality clashes aren't legitimate patient care concerns. In the event of a lawsuit, the plaintiff's lawyer will exploit conflicts among codefendants.
   Instead of documenting these problems, talk with your nurse-manager or consult with the practitioner directly if an order puzzles you. If another nurse writes personal accusations or charges of incompetence in a medical record, talk to nurse about the implications of doing this. Remember, you're responsible for your actions.

3. Don't mention incident reports
Incident reports are confidential and filed separately from the patient's medical record. Document only the facts of an incident in the medical record, and never write *incident report* or indicate that you filed one.
   Keep in mind that incident reports may be discoverable depending on which state you practice in. This means that the plaintiff's attorney may have access to them depending on state laws.

4. Don't use words associated with errors
Terms like *by mistake, accidentally, somehow, unintentionally, miscalculated,* and *confusing* are bonus words to the plaintiff's attorney. Steer clear of words that suggest an error was made or a patient's safety was jeopardized. Let the facts speak for themselves.

5. Don't name a second patient
Naming a second patient in a patient's medical record violates confidentiality. Instead, write *roommate,* the patient's initials, or the room and bed number.

6. Don't document casual conversations with colleagues
Telling your nurse-manager or a practitioner in the elevator or restroom about a patient's deteriorating condition doesn't qualify as informing. In these types of conversations, the person you are talking to may not even realize you expect an intervention. When notifying someone, clearly state *why* you're notifying the person and focus on the facts so that appropriate action can be taken. Otherwise, you can't document that you informed anyone.

liable. Be familiar with your facility's discharge processes and know your responsibilities with this very important process.
   Many facilities give patients printed instruction sheets that describe treatments and home care procedures. Make sure your patient can read English before giving printed instruction sheets; if not, provide the instructions in the language the patient can understand if possible and utilize a qualified interpreter, such as a language line, to

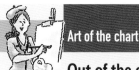

Art of the chart

Out of the ordinary

This note shows the right way to chart atypical information.

2/18/2017	0600	Pt found sitting on floor next to bed. Pt awake and oriented. States "I was getting up to go to the bathroom." Pt denies pain. No injury noted. Pt states "I slid to the ground when my knees gave out." B/P 144/86, HR 105, RR 16, Pox 94%. Pt assisted back to bed and made comfortable. Call light within reach. Bed in low position. ——————— C. Cashman RN
2/18/2017	0630	Dr. M. Steiger notified regarding fall. No orders given. House supervisor also notified. ——————— C. Cashman RN

discuss the instructions with the patient and family. Be sure to follow your facility's policies on use of language interpretation and documentation requirements. In court, these materials may be used as evidence that instruction took place. To support testimony, they should be tailored to each patient's specific needs and contain any verbal or written instructions you provided. Some facilities require that a signed copy of the discharge instructions be placed in the medical record as proof that the patient or family received the instructions.

Documentation of referrals to home health care agencies or other community providers is another essential component of discharge planning. This is often completed by a case manager, who has a better understanding of the documentation requirements. With inadequate documentation, a home health claim can be denied.

When to document

Finding time to document can be difficult during a busy shift. However, the timeliness of entries is a major issue in malpractice suits.

Don't get ahead of yourself

Document nursing care when you perform it or shortly afterward. Never document ahead of time—your notes will be inaccurate, and

Understanding negligence

Inadequate observation of patients that leads to misdiagnosis or injury is a common cause of lawsuits involving nurses. Most of these lawsuits involve issues of negligence—the failure to exercise the degree of care that a person of ordinary prudence would exercise under the same circumstances. A claim of negligence requires that there be a duty owed by one person to another, that the duty be breached, and that injury resulted.

Malpractice is a more restricted, specialized type of negligence that applies to professionals and is defined as a violation of professional duty to act with reasonable care and in good faith. Several states have begun to recognize nursing negligence as a form of malpractice.

Avoid negligence cases by documenting any and all unusual patient events.

Case in point

The trouble with charting by exception

The case of *Lama v. Borras* (1994) shows the importance of thoroughly documenting assessment findings.

"Back" ground
The patient underwent disc surgery for which prophylactic antibiotics weren't ordered. Postoperatively, the patient started to show signs of infection, including "very bloody" dressings and pain at the incision site. Ultimately, the patient was diagnosed with discitis (an infection of the space in-between discs) and was given antibiotics. The patient was hospitalized for several months while undergoing treatment for the infection.

Exception = incomplete
Details regarding the patient's infection symptoms weren't known because the facility's nurses were instructed to "chart by exception," a system in which nurses don't record qualitative observations at each shift; rather, they record such observations only when it's deemed necessary to document important changes in the patient's condition. It was alleged that the nurses' failure to report the patient's symptoms during each nursing shift caused the late detection of the patient's infection.

The verdict
The court stated there was evidence to suggest that charting by exception didn't regularly record information important to an infection diagnosis, such as the changing characteristics of the surgical wound and the patient's complaints of postoperative pain. One of the attending nurses conceded that under the charting by exception policy, she wouldn't report a patient's pain if she didn't administer medicine or if she gave the patient only an aspirin-type medication. The court also concluded that the intermittent documentation of possible signs of infection failed to record the sort of continuous danger signals that would most likely spur early intervention by a practitioner.

you'll leave out information about the patient's response to treatment. This is also considered falsification, contributes to errors, confusion, and is a patient safety concern. Even if you did what you charted, a lawyer might ask, "Do you occasionally chart something before doing it?" If you answer "yes," the jury won't see the chart as a reliable indicator of what you actually did, which destroys your credibility. (See *Documenting ahead*, page 132.)

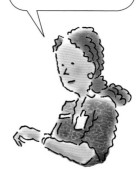

Document ahead of time? Never! My credibility is at stake.

Who should document

State NPAs have strict rules about who can document. Breaking these rules can cause your state board to take actions against your nursing license.

Documenting ahead

In the case of *Beene v. St. Vincent Mercy Medical* Center (2000), a court upheld a hospital's disciplinary suspension of a nurse after the death of a patient under her care. The patient had a heart attack, but no audible alarm was sounded when the patient went into arrest because the alarms on the cardiac monitor were disengaged. During the subsequent investigation, it was discovered that the nurse noted on the patient's medical chart that the alarms were active at 4:00 p.m., 5:00 p.m., and 6:00 p.m.; however, the patient was already dead at these times. The nurse admitted that to save time, she had made all entries regarding the alarms at the beginning of her shift rather than at hourly intervals as suggested on the medical chart. The nurse attempted to establish that it was common practice for nurses to "document ahead" or mark hourly intervals 3 or 4 hours before treatment is administered. The court found that documenting ahead was a violation of hospital policy and, in the circumstances of the case, the action amounted to falsifying medical records.

Finish what you started

No matter how busy you are, never ask another nurse to complete your documentation (and never complete another nurse's documentation). Doing so is a dangerous practice that may be specifically prohibited by your state's NPA. If the other nurse makes an error or misinterprets information, the patient can be harmed. Then if the patient sues you for negligence, both you and your facility will be held accountable because delegated documentation doesn't meet nursing standards.

Delegating documentation has another consequence: It destroys the credibility and value of the medical record both in the facility and in court. Judges give little, if any, weight to medical records containing secondhand observations or hearsay evidence.

Risk management and documentation

A health care facility's reputation for safe, reliable, and effective service is its main defense against liability claims. Well-coordinated risk management and quality management programs show the public that the facility is being managed in a legally responsible manner. If complaints arise, a good program ensures that they're handled promptly to contain the damage and minimize liability claims. (See *Understanding the roles of risk management and quality management*, page 133.)

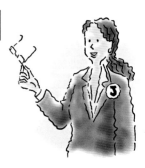

Understanding the roles of risk management and quality management

Think of it like this, when a patient is harmed as a result of a medical error, risk management usually conducts an in-depth investigation to evaluate liability exposure to the organization so that future losses can be prevented. Quality management's primary goal is to improve the quality of care by designing formal process improvement initiatives that target underlying causes of an event.

Two for one

Many facilities combine these two programs into their educational efforts. They place a high priority on teaching medical residents, nurses, and practitioners about malpractice claims, staff members' reporting obligations, proper informational and reporting channels, and principles of risk management and quality management.

In addition, TJC requires health care facilities to identify and manage sentinel events. A sentinel event is a patient safety event that affects a patient and results in any of the following:

- death
- permanent harm
- severe temporary harm and intervention is required to sustain life.

When an organization suspects an undesirable event, it's required to initiate an intense analysis of the situation to determine the root cause and place systems/processes into place to prevent the same event from occurring in the future.

Some events which would be considered sentinel by TJC may include:

- inpatient suicide or up to 72 hours after discharge
- confirmed transfusion reaction
- surgical/invasive procedure on wrong patients, wrong site, or wrong procedure
- unintended retention of a foreign object after an invasive procedure.

Mining the records for potential risk

Sometimes, documentation reveals potential problems within a health care facility. For example, documentation might reveal that a certain procedure repeatedly leads to patient injury or another type of accident. Risk management programs help reduce injuries and accidents, minimize financial loss, and meet the guidelines of TJC and other regulatory agencies.

In the past, the focuses of risk management and quality management departments were to maintain and improve facilities and equipment and ensure employee, visitor, and patient safety. Today, the focus is on identifying, evaluating, and reducing patient injury in specialty units that have the greatest malpractice risks.

Preventing adverse events

Risk management has three main goals:
1. decreasing the number of claims by promptly identifying and following up on adverse events (early warning systems)
2. reducing the frequency of preventable injuries and accidents leading to lawsuits by maintaining or improving the quality of care
3. controlling costs related to claims by pinpointing trouble spots early and working with the patient and family.

Early warning systems

Early warning systems can pinpoint much useful information. However, to be effective, they need:
*   a strong organizational structure
*   cooperation between risk management and quality management departments
*   commitment of all staff members to report adverse events to their supervisor so that the medical records can be reviewed and/or the staff member involved can be interviewed. Based on information collected, next actions are determined, which may include remedial education, monitoring, or restricted privileges.
*   commitment of key staff members—such as nurses, practitioners, administrators, and chiefs of high-risk services—to analyze the information
*   commitment of all staff members to be compliant with policies and procedures in order to maintain and maximize quality patient care. The most commonly used early warning systems are *incident reporting* and *occurrence screening*.

Reporting the out of the ordinary

An incident or occurrence report refers to the documentation of events that are inconsistent with a health care facility's ordinary routine, regardless of whether injury occurs. Practitioner, nurses, or other staff are responsible for reporting such events when they're observed or shortly afterward. Examples include a patient fall, the unplanned return of a patient to the operating room, or a medication error.

Let's review

Occurrence screening involves reviewing medical records to find adverse events. Both general indicators of adverse events (such as a nosocomial infection or medication error) and more specific indicators (such as an incorrect sponge count during surgery) are considered.

Reducing injuries and accidents

Many health care facilities coordinate educational efforts to help prevent injuries and accidents that may lead to lawsuits.

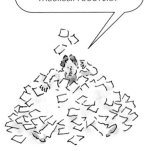

Occurrence screening requires careful review of medical records.

Making sure everyone is on the same page

The facility may reach out to a specific employee, such as a nurse or practitioner, who has been identified as having a particular problem, or to a larger population, such as new nurses or residents, that may face the same types of problems. Required teaching topics for new employees include malpractice claims, reporting obligations, proper informational and reporting channels, and principles of risk management and quality management.

Cost control

Systematic, well-coordinated risk management and quality management programs demonstrate to the public that the facility is managed in a legally responsible way. When complaints do arise, risk managers handle them promptly to contain the damage and minimize liability claims.

Managing incidents

Despite risk management programs, adverse events still occur. Health care facilities rely on the following sources to identify dangerous situations or trends:

- *Incident reports*, also called *occurrence reports*, can be a primary source of information for lawyers. Lawyers use the reports when researching potential lawsuits and in court as evidence. In some states, incident reports, under the law, may not be allowed to be accessed or are not "discoverable" by the plaintiff's attorney in a lawsuit. Become familiar with your state laws regarding incident reports. Also, do not provide copies of incident reports to anyone, unless directed by risk management.
- *Nurses* are usually the first ones to recognize potential problems because they spend so much time with patients and families. They know which patients are dissatisfied with their care and which ones have complications that may lead to injuries. If such a situation arises, nurse-managers or administrators may become involved to initiate specific "customer service" actions to help resolve a problem before it worsens.
- *Patient-representatives* keep files of patient complaints, identify litigious patients, and maintain contact with the patient and family after an incident has occurred.
- *The business office and medical records department* may be alerted to potential lawsuits when a patient threatens to sue after receiving the facility bill or when a patient or a lawyer requests a copy of the medical record.

- *Other sources* can also help. For example, the engineering department has information on the safety of the hospital environment; purchasing, biomedical engineering, and the pharmacy can report on the safety and adequacy of products and equipment; and social workers, hospital clergy, volunteers, and patient escorts commonly know about highly dissatisfied patients. *Remember:* Whenever you get a report from one of these sources, request that the person reporting the problem document it thoroughly in the patient's medical record and fill out an incident report.

> *Other members of the health care team can provide information to help manage incidents.*

The claim chain reaction

Once the risk manager learns of a potential or actual lawsuit, facility's processes should be followed to notify the appropriate parties which may include: insurance company, practitioners or staff involved, and the facility's defense attorney. If the medical record is still on paper, the medical records department should be notified so that the record can be copied and the original stored in a safe place to prevent tampering. Now that most facilities have gone to paperless records or EHRs, this process is usually no longer necessary.

A claim notice should also trigger a peer review of the medical record. This review measures the practitioner's conduct against the professional standards of conduct for the particular situation. This information is used by the risk manager and the facility's attorney to investigate the claim's merit, the facility's responsibility, and areas where changes are needed. The standard required for a successful defense isn't always as high as the facility's optimal standard.

Eight legal hazards

Every day, you face patient care situations that could land you in court. Your challenge is to watch out for potential pitfalls and know how to document them defensively when they arise. This section describes eight volatile legal situations.

Hazard #1: Incident reports

Whenever you witness an adverse event, file an incident report. Some things to report are injuries from restraints, burns, or other causes; falls (even if the patient wasn't injured); medication error; and a patient's insistence on being discharged against medical advice (AMA). If an incident report form doesn't leave enough space to fully describe an incident, attach an additional page of comments. (See *Completing an incident report*, page 137.)

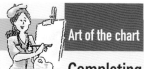

Art of the chart

Completing an incident report

When you witness a reportable event, you must fill out an incident report. Many facilities have gone to electronic incident reporting systems; however, most include the following pertinent information.

INCIDENT REPORT

Name *Greta Manning*
Address *7 Worth Way, Boston, MA*
Phone *(617) 555-1122*

9. DATE OF INCIDENT	10. TIME OF INCIDENT
3-14-2017	1442

11. EXACT LOCATION OF INCIDENT (Bldg., Floor, Room No., Area)
4-Main, Rm. 447

Addressograph if patient

12. TYPE OF INCIDENT (CHECK ONE ONLY) ☐ PATIENT ☐ EMPLOYEE ☑ VISITOR ☐ VOLUNTEER ☐ OTHER _____ (Specify)

13. DESCRIPTION OF THE INCIDENT (WHO, WHAT, WHEN, WHERE, HOW, WHY) (Use Back of Form if Necessary)

Wife of pt found on floor next to left side of bed. States "I was trying to put the siderail of the bed down to sit on my husband's bed and I fell down."

> State only what you saw or heard.

> Describe relevant conditions.

14. FLOOR CONDITIONS ☐ OTHER _____ ☑ CLEAN & SMOOTH ☐ SLIPPERY (WET)   FRAME OF BED ☑ LOW ☐ HIGH   NIGHT LIGHT ☐ YES ☑ NO

15. WERE BED RAILS PRESENT? ☐ NO ☐ 1 UP ☑ 2 UP ☐ 3 UP ☐ 4 UP   17. OTHER RESTRAINTS (TYPE & EXTENT) *N/A*

18. AMBULATION PRIVILEGE ☐ UNLIMITED ☐ LIMITED WITH ASSISTANCE ☐ COMPLETE BEDREST ☐ OTHER

19. WAS NARCOTICS, ANALGESICS, HYPNOTICS, SEDATIVES, DIURETICS, ANTIHYPERTENSIVES OR ANTICONVULSANTS GIVEN DURING LAST 4 HOURS? ☐ YES ☑ NO

DRUG | AMOUNT | TIME

PATIENT INCIDENTS

20. PHYSICIAN NOTIFIED NAME OF PHYSICIAN *J. Reynolds, MD* | DATE *3-14-2017* | TIME | COMPLETE IF APPLICABLE *1445*

EMPLOYEE INCIDENTS

21. DEPARTMENT | 22. JOB TITLE | 23. SOCIAL SECURITY #

24. MARITAL STATUS

27. SUPERVISOR NOTIFIED NAME OF SUPERVISOR *C. Jones, RN* DATE *3-14-2017* TIME *1500* | 28. LOCATION (WHERE TREATMENT WAS RENDERED)

29. NAME, ADDRESS AND TELEPHONE NUMBER OF WITNESS(ES) OR PERSONS FAMILIAR WITH INCIDENT - WITNESS OR NOT
Connie Smith, RN (617)555-0912 1 Main St., Boston, MA

ALL INCIDENTS

SIGNATURE OF PERSON PREPARING REPORT *Connie Smith* | TITLE *RN* | 31. DATE OF REPORT *3-14-2017*

> List the name, telephone number, and address of anyone involved.

To be completed for all cases involving injury or illness (DO NOT USE ABBREVIATIONS) (Use back of Form if necessary)

...nt in Emergency Department after reported fall in husband's room. 12 cm x 12 cm ...ea noted on right hip. X-rays negative for fracture. Good range of motion. no c/o ...O. Ice pack applied. —— J. Reynolds, MD

33. DISPOSITION
sent home, written instructions provided to pt and wife; pt and wife verbalized understanding of instructions.

34. PERSON NOTIFIED OTHER THAN HOSPITAL PERSONNEL NAME AND ADDRESS *R.Manning (daughter) address same as pt* | 35. DATE *3-14-2017* | 36. TIME *1500*

37. PHYSICIAN'S SIGNATURE *J. Reynolds, MD* | 38. DATE *3-14-2017*

The form's function

An incident report has two functions:

1. It informs the facility's administration of the incident so the risk management staff can work on preventing similar incidents.
2. It alerts the facility's administration and insurance company to a potential claim and the need for further investigation.

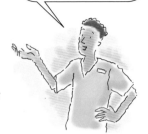

Following the guidelines here will reduce your legal risks.

It's an eyewitness report

Only people who witnessed an incident should fill out and sign an incident report, and each witness should file a separate report. After the report is filed, it may be reviewed by the nurse-manager, the practitioner who examined the patient after the incident, various department heads and administrators, the facility's attorney, and the insurance company.

Because incident reports will be read by many people and may even turn up in court, you must follow strict guidelines when completing them. (See *Tips for reporting incidents.*)

Facilities are continually revising their incident report forms; some are now computerized, which permits classifying and counting incidents to indicate trends, as well as creating the ability of sending the report to several people at the same time.

Advice from the experts

Tips for reporting incidents

In the past, a plaintiff's lawyer wasn't permitted to see incident reports. Today, however, many states allow lawyers access to incident reports if they make their requests through proper channels. So, when completing an incident report, keep in mind who may read it and follow these guidelines:

• Include essential information and stick to the facts, such as the identity of the person involved in the incident, the exact time and place of the incident, and the name of the practitioner you notified.

• Document any unusual occurrences that you witnessed.

• Record the events and the consequences for the patient in enough detail that administrators can decide whether or not to investigate further.

• Write objectively, avoiding opinions, judgments, conclusions, or assumptions about who or what caused the incident. Tell your opinions to your supervisor, nurse-manager, or the risk manager privately at a later time.

• Describe only what you saw and heard and the actions you took to provide care at the scene. Unless you saw a patient fall, write *Found pt lying on the floor.*

• Don't admit that you're at fault or blame someone else. Steer clear of statements such as *Better staffing would have prevented this incident.*

• Don't offer suggestions about how to prevent the incident from happening again.

• Don't include detailed statements from witnesses and descriptions of remedial action; these are normally part of an investigative follow-up.

• Don't put the report in the medical record. Send it to the person designated to review it according to your facility's policy.

• Never document in the medical record that you completed an incident report.

Documenting incidents in progress notes

When documenting an incident in the medical record, follow these guidelines:

- Write a factual account of the incident, including assessments, treatments, and follow-up care as well as the patient's response. This account shows that the patient was appropriately assessed and treated and then closely monitored after the incident. Make sure the descriptions in the medical record match those in the incident report.
- Don't write *incident report completed* after documenting the event. This destroys the confidential nature of the report and may result in a lawsuit. For the same reason, the practitioner shouldn't write an order for an incident report in the medical record.
- In documenting the incident, include everything the patient or family member says about the patient's role in the incident. For example, you might write *Pt stated, "The nurse told me to ask for help before I went to the bathroom, but I decided to go on my own."* In a negligence lawsuit, this information may help the defense lawyer show that the incident was entirely or partially the patient's fault. If the jury finds that the patient was partially at fault, the concept of *contributory negligence* may be used to reduce or even eliminate the patient's recovery of damages.

Hazard #2: Informed consent

A patient must sign a consent form before most treatments and procedures. Informed consent means that the patient understands the proposed therapy and its risks and agrees to proceed with the treatment or procedure. The practitioner performing the procedure or treatment is legally responsible for explaining the procedure and its risks, benefits, and alternatives prior to the procedure or treatment being performed. However, the practitioner may ask you to witness the patient's signature. Some facilities may specifically require the person who informs the patient of the treatment or procedure to be the one to obtain the consent. Check with your facility's legal counsel if you have any questions. (See *Sign here: Witnessing a consent form,* page 140.)

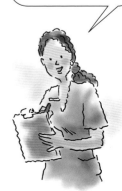

In the form, state the name of the practitioner performing the procedure and not just the group that the practitioner may be a part of.

Waive it good-bye

The legal requirement for obtaining informed consent can be waived only if:

- a mentally competent patient states a wish to not know the details of a treatment or procedure
- an urgent medical or surgical situation occurs (many facilities specify how you should document such an emergency).

Most facilities use a standard consent form that lists the legal requirements for consent. If the patient doesn't understand the practitioner's explanation or asks for more information, answer all

Sign here: Witnessing a consent form

After the practitioner informs the patient about a medical procedure or treatment, an order may be written for you to obtain the patient's consent—obtaining the patient's signature on the consent form and then signing as a witness. Before doing so, review this checklist:

• Make sure that the patient is competent, awake, alert, oriented, and aware. The patient should not be under the influence of alcohol, illicit drugs, or prescribed medications that will impair patient's understanding or judgment.

• Ask the patient whether the practitioner explained the diagnosis, proposed procedure or treatment, expected outcome, and answered any questions presented. Also ask whether the patient understood all that was said.

• Ask the patient whether the risks and benefits of the treatment or procedure were discussed, as well as the possible consequences of refusing it, and alternative treatments or procedures.

• Ask the patient about any concerns or questions about the procedure or treatment. If so, help the patient obtain answers from the practitioner or other appropriate sources prior to you and the patient signing the consent.

• Tell the patient that the procedure or treatment may be refused without having other care or support withdrawn and that the patient can withdraw consent after giving it.

• Notify your nurse-manager and the practitioner immediately if you suspect that the patient has doubts about the treatment or procedure, hasn't been properly informed, or has been coerced into giving consent. Performing a treatment or procedure without voluntary consent may be considered battery.

• Objectively document your assessment of the patient's understanding in the medical record, noting the situation, patient responses, and the actions you took.

• When you're satisfied that the patient is well informed, have the patient sign the consent form including the date and time and then sign your name as a witness.

• Remember that you're responsible for obtaining verbal informed consent for any procedures that you'll be performing, such as inserting an intravenous (I.V.) catheter or a urinary catheter, even though a general treatment consent was signed upon admission.

questions that fall within the scope of your practice. Be sure to document your interaction with the patient. (See *Informed consent*, page 141.)

Hazard #3: Advance directives

The Patient Self-Determination Act requires health care facilities to provide information about the patient's right to choose and refuse treatment. Facilities must also ask patients whether they have advance directives, which are documents that state a patient's wishes regarding life-sustaining medical care in case the patient is no longer able to communicate wishes regarding care. Your job is to document that the patient received the required information and whether or not the patient brought a copy of the advance directive to the health care facility. (See *Tips for dealing with advance directives*, page 142.) Facility policies and state laws vary, so make sure you know what's required in your state and facility. A patient may have established end-of-life medical

Art of the chart

Informed consent

A patient's signature on a consent form implies understanding the risks, benefits, alternatives, and consequences of refusal of a procedure and agreeing to undergo it. Here's a typical form. Keep in mind that some facilities have electronic informed consents built into their EHRs.

CONSENT FOR OPERATION AND RENDERING OF OTHER MEDICAL SERVICES

1. I hereby authorize Dr. _____Wesley_____ to perform upon _____Joseph Smith_____ (Patient name), the following surgical and/or medical procedures: (State specific nature of the procedures to be performed) _____Exploratomy laparotomy_____

2. I understand that the procedure(s) will be p_____ or under the supervision of Dr. _____Wesley_____, who is authorized to utilize the services of o_____ use staff as he or she deems necessary or advisable.

   > The name of the physician performing the procedure needs to be on the form—not just the group that the practitioner is a part of.

   > The form should state the specific procedure under consideration. Abbreviations for the procedure are not acceptable. It must be written out entirely.

   ____ed to me that during th_____ en conditions may be revealed that necessitate _____ original procedure(s) o_____ set forth in Paragraph 1, I therefore authorize and ____ve named doctor, and his or her associates or assistants, perform such medical surgical procedures as are ____able in the exercise of professional judgment.

   ____ure and purpose of the procedure(s), possible alternative methods of diagnosis or treatment, the risks ____lity of complications, and the consequences of the procedure(s). I acknowledge that no guarantee or assur-____e as to the results that may be obtained.

   > The patient acknowledges understanding and its risks and agrees to undergo it.

5. I authorize the above named doctor to administer local or regional anesthesia (for a_____ement a separate consent must be signed by the patient or patient's authorized representative).

6. I understand that if it is necessary for me to receive a blood transfusion during this _____zation, the blood will be supplied by sources available to the hospital and tested in accordance with _____ations. I understand that there are risks in transfusion, including but not limited to allergic, febrile, _____ reactions, and the transmission of infectious diseases, such as hepatitis and AIDS (Acquired Immune Deficiency Syndrome). I hereby consent to blood transfusion(s) and blood derivative(s).

7. I hereby authorize representatives from Valley Medical Center to photograph or videotape me for the purpose of research or medical education. It is understood and agreed that patient confidentiality shall be preserved.

8. I authorize the doctor named above and his or her associates and assistants and Valley Medical Center to preserve for scientific purposes or to dispose of any tissue, organs, or other body parts removed during surgery or other diagnostic procedures in accordance with customary medical practice.

9. I certify that I have read and fully understand the above consent statement. In addition, I have been afforded an opportunity to ask whatever questions I might have regarding the procedure(s) to be performed and they have been answered to my satisfaction.

_____Joseph Smith_____   _____C. Gurney, RN_____   _____03/15/2017_____
Legal Patient or Authorized Representative   Witness   Date
(State Relationship to Patient)

> Signing indicates only that you're witnessing the patient's signature.

If the patient is unable to consent on his or her own behalf, complete the following:

Patient _____ is unable to consent because _____

_____

_____   _____M. Wesley, MD_____   _____03/15/2017_____
Legally Responsible Person   Practitioner   Date

Tips for dealing with advance directives

Many patients wait until they're hospitalized to consider an advance directive or to make significant legal decisions. So, be prepared to offer information and advice and to record the patient's wishes in a legally appropriate manner. Here are some important points to remember.

Legal competence

Only a competent adult can execute a legally binding document. To prevent a patient's relatives from raising questions about competence later, discuss the patient's mental status with the practitioner and, possibly, a psychiatrist, if indicated. Be sure to document the patient's mental status assessment in the medical record before the patient signs any legal documents.

Living will and durable power of attorney

If a patient has a living will or durable power of attorney for health care, a copy should be obtained and placed into the medical record. Also, you should know how to contact the person with decision-making power. If the patient doesn't have the document on admission, ask a family member to bring it to the health care facility. As your patient's advocate, you must ensure that the wishes

of the patient are properly executed. If conflicts arise, discuss them with your nurse-manager as well as with a risk manager.

If a patient wants to execute a living will during the hospital stay, you aren't required, or even allowed in some states, to sign as a witness. Many facilities have the social service or risk management department that oversee this process. Find out who is responsible in your facility. The person who acts as witness can be held accountable for the patient's competence. Place the signed and witnessed document in the chart.

Last will and testament

In some facilities, dictating a patient's last will and testament is so commonplace that special forms have been designed for it. If this situation occurs often in your facility and you do not have appropriate forms, discuss creating a form with your manager.

If no form exists in your facility, and a patient wants to dictate a last will and testament to you, document the request and what has been done to facilitate it—for example, who has been contacted and when. Become familiar with your facility's processes and be sure to follow them.

treatment care via the use of Physician Orders for Life-Sustaining Treatment (POLST) and not by completing an advanced directive. If a patient is admitted and has a POLST form, the practitioner is legally bound to follow the orders already in place, unless the patient states otherwise. (See *What is POLST?*)

What is POLST?

POLST is a national program (the National POLST Paradigm) established to provide seriously ill patients with portable physician orders indicating resuscitation wishes. The physician, along with the patient, completes the specific National POLST Paradigm form, which contains a set of medical orders, similar to "do-not-resuscitate" (DNR) orders. It is not an advance directive and does not assign health care power of attorney. This form is easily recognizable (bright pink) and must be honored when presented to a health care facility. Other names for this program (implemented per individual state) include medical orders for life-sustaining treatment (MOLST), medical orders for scope of treatment (MOST), and physician orders for scope of treatment (POST).

A change may be in order

When a patient's advance directive is given to the practitioner, orders may be provided based on the patient's wishes. For example, if the patient's family submits an advance directive that includes the information that the patient doesn't want to be resuscitated, a DNR order may be written.

A DNR order can be changed at any time if the patient requests. (See *Documenting last wishes*.)

Who else can give a DNR order?

If the patient doesn't request a DNR status, or if no policies exist, the practitioner may write the order if it's medically appropriate and the patient understands the impact of the DNR order. If the patient is incompetent, an appropriate surrogate must give consent for the practitioner to write the DNR order.

Advice from the experts

Documenting last wishes

Because do-not-resuscitate (DNR) orders are legally recognized, you won't incur liability if you don't attempt to resuscitate a patient with a DNR order and that patient later dies. You may, however, incur liability if you initiate resuscitation on a patient who has a DNR order. Every patient with a DNR order should have a written order on file. But if a patient doesn't have a DNR order, you're obligated to attempt resuscitation if the situation warrants it.

How should you proceed?

If a terminally ill patient without a DNR order requests to not be resuscitated in a crisis, document the patient's wishes along with the patient's degree of awareness and orientation. Then contact the practitioner and your nurse-manager, and ask for assistance from administration, legal services, or social services. Don't place yourself in the middle. Let the practitioner and the patient's family make the decisions.

If the practitioner knows about the patient's wishes but still refuses to write a DNR order, document this information in your notes. Like you, the practitioner must abide by the patient's wishes and may be found liable by not following the wishes. If the patient has prepared an advance directive, make sure the practitioner has seen it. For issues that cannot be resolved, some facilities have implemented ethics committees to help deal with these situations.

A patient's right

The patient has the right to change advance directives at any time. Because the patient's requests may differ from what the family or practitioner wants, document discrepancies carefully. Use social services or the legal department for advice on how to proceed. (See *Check this out: Advance directive checklist*, page 145.)

Two common types of advance directives are living will and durable power of attorney for health care.

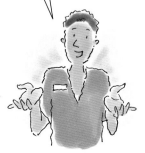

When the patient's wishes about life-sustaining care clash with the practitioner's or family members', document the discrepancy.

Living will

In making a living will, a legally competent person specifically declares what medical care is desired or not desired if experiencing a terminal illness. Living wills may apply only to treatment decisions made after a terminally ill patient becomes comatose and has no reasonable chance of recovery. They usually authorize the practitioner to withhold or discontinue lifesaving measures.

State-ments

Most states recognize living wills as valid legal documents. Although the legal requirements vary from state to state, most states specify:
- circumstances under which a living will applies
- who is authorized to make a living will (usually only competent adults)
- limitations or restrictions on care that can be refused (e.g., some states don't allow refusal of food and water)
- elements the will must contain to be considered a legal document, including witnessing requirements
- who is immune from liability for following a living will's directions
- procedure for rescinding a living will.

Durable power of attorney

A durable power of attorney for health care enables a person to state what type of care desired or not desired and names another person to make health care choices if the patient becomes legally incompetent. This person is usually a family member or friend or, in rare instances, the practitioner.

Hazard #4: Patients who refuse treatment

You're also responsible for helping patients make informed decisions about continuing treatment. When treatment is refused, important patient care, safety, and documentation issues come into play.

Refusing treatment

Any mentally competent adult can legally refuse treatment after being fully informed about the medical condition and the likely

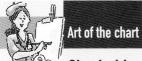

Art of the chart

Check this out: Advance directive checklist

The Joint Commission requires that information on advance directives be charted on the admission assessment form. However, many facilities have built checklists into their electronic documentation system. Below is an example of checklist elements.

ADVANCE DIRECTIVE CHECKLIST

Check appropriate boxes.

I. DISTRIBUTION OF ADVANCE DIRECTIVE INFORMATION

   A. Advance directive information was presented to the patient: .... ☑

      1. At the time of preadmission testing .... ☑

      2. Upon inpatient admission.. ☐

      3. Interpretive services contacted.. ☐

      4. Information was read to the patient .... ☐

   B. Advance directive information was presented to the next of kin as the patient is incapacitated.. ☐

   C. Advance directive information was not distributed as the patient is incapacitated and no relative or next of kin was available. .... ☐

Mary Barren, RN   *03/15/2017*
RN   **DATE**

II. ASSESSMENT OF ADVANCE DIRECTIVE UPON ADMISSION

	Upon admission		Upon transfer to Critical Care Unit	
	YES	NO	YES	NO

   A. Does the patient have an advance directive?

      If yes, was the attending physician notified?

	Upon admission		Upon transfer	
A. Does the patient have an advance directive?	☐	☑	☐	☐
If yes, was the attending physician notified?	☐		☐	

   B. If no advance directive, does the patient want to execute an advance directive?

      If yes, was the attending physician notified?

      Was the patient referred to resources?

	Upon admission		Upon transfer	
B. If no advance directive, does the patient want to execute an advance directive?	☑	☐	☐	☐
If yes, was the attending physician notified?	☑		☐	
Was the patient referred to resources?	☑		☐	

Sign and date.

Mary Barren, RN
RN   RN
03/15/2017
DATE   DATE

III. RECEIPT OF AN ADVANCE DIRECTIVE AFTER ADMISSION

   A. The patient has presented an advance directive after admission, and the attending physician has been notified.

Sign here if the patient brought an advance directive and presented it after admission.

RN   **DATE**

consequences of refusal. Thus, refusal can include mechanical ventilation, tube feedings, antibiotics, fluids, and other treatments that are needed to keep the patient alive.

The patient who says "no"

When your patient refuses treatment, document the patient's exact words. Inform the patient of the risks involved in refusing treatment, preferably in writing. If the patient still refuses treatment, document that you didn't provide the prescribed treatment and then notify the practitioner. The practitioner will explain the risks to the patient again. If treatment is still refused, the patient may be asked by practitioner to sign a refusal-of-treatment release form, which you may need to sign as a witness. (See *Witnessing refusal of treatment*.)

If the patient won't sign this form, document this, also. For extra protection, your facility may require you to have the patient's spouse or closest relative sign another refusal-of-treatment release form.

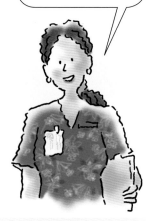

When a patient refuses treatment, document the patient's exact words.

Art of the chart

Witnessing refusal of treatment

To prevent misunderstandings and lawsuits if a patient refuses treatment, the practitioner must explain the risks involved in making this choice. If the patient still refuses treatment, the practitioner will ask the patient to sign a refusal-of-treatment release form, such as the one below, which you may need to witness.

The patient acknowledges that he understands the risks of refusing treatment.

REFUSAL-OF-TREATMENT RELEASE FORM

I, ___Joseph Arden___, refuse to allow anyone to ___administer parenteral nutrition___.
   (patient's name)   (insert treatment)

The risks attendant to my refusal have been fully explained to me, and I fully understand the benefits of this treatment. I also understand that my refusal of treatment seriously reduces my chances for regaining normal health and may endanger my life.

I hereby release ___Memorial General___, its nurses and employees, together with all doctors in any way connected
                (name of facility)
with me as a patient, from liability for respecting and following my express wishes and direction.

___Donna Burns, RN___   ___Joseph Arden___
(Witness's signature)   (Patient's or legal guardian's signature)

___2/17/2017___   ___76___
(Date)   (Patient's age)

Get to them early

More and more facilities are informing patients soon after admission about their future treatment options. Discuss the patient's wishes at your first opportunity, and document the discussion in case the patient becomes incompetent later. It may be helpful to use a chaplain or someone from social services to speak with the patient to verify specific wishes.

Legal guidelines

Failure to respond appropriately to a patient's refusal to accept treatment may have serious legal consequences. To prevent problems, take these steps:

- Confirm the patient's condition and prognosis with the practitioner and record them in the medical record.
- Make sure that the practitioner documented the patient's understanding of the consequences of the refusal, such as pain or decreased life expectancy or quality of life.
- Search the medical record for a living will or a durable power of attorney for health care.
- Search the medical record for documentation of conversations between the patient and health care providers, including the conversation about the patient's final decision to withhold treatment. Documentation should include the dates of conversations, the full names of people involved, the circumstances, and what treatments and medical conditions were discussed.
- DNR orders should be reviewed every 48 to 72 hours or according to your facility's policy.
- DNR orders must be written and signed by the practitioner; they can't be provided as verbal orders or telephone orders.
- Refuse written or spoken orders for "slow codes," such as calling the practitioner before resuscitating a patient, doing cardiopulmonary resuscitation (CPR) but withholding drugs, giving oxygen but withholding CPR, or not putting a patient on a ventilator. These orders are unethical and illegal.
- Suggest that your facility set up an ethics committee to resolve problems about withholding treatment.

Hazard #5: Documenting for unlicensed personnel

Anyone reading your documentation assumes this information is a firsthand account of care provided—unless you document otherwise. In some settings, nursing assistants and technicians aren't allowed to make formal entries to the medical record. In such cases, determine what care was provided, assess the patient and the task performed (e.g., a dressing change), and document your findings. Be sure to record the full names and titles of unlicensed personnel who provided care. Don't just record their initials.

Countersign-language

If your facility allows unlicensed personnel to document, you may have to countersign their documentation. If your facility's policy states that the unlicensed person must provide care in your presence, don't countersign unless you actually witness the actions provided. If the policy states that you don't have to be there, your countersigning indicates that the documentation describes care that other people had the authority and competence to perform and that you verified that the procedures were performed. You can specifically document that you reviewed the documentation and consulted with the technician on certain aspects of care. Of course, you must document any follow-up care you provide.

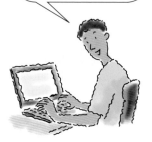

If you're documenting care provided by unlicensed personnel, assess the patient and the task performed and document your findings.

Hazard #6: Using restraints

When physical restraints are ordered for a patient, you have several responsibilities, including:
- documenting the reason for the restraints and any alternative interventions provided to alter patient behavior and avoid use of restraints
- notifying the practitioner and obtaining an order for the restraints
- applying the restraints appropriately to prevent harm
- ensuring that the patient's dignity and safety are maintained
- monitoring the patient for problems associated with the restraints
- performing range-of-motion exercises on all extremities at regular intervals
- making sure the patient has access to the call signal
- assessing the patient's vital signs, circulation status, hydration and elimination needs, level of distress and agitation, mental status, cognitive functioning, and skin integrity
- teaching the patient and family the reason for the restraints and the criteria for release (if able)
- assessing if the patient has met criteria for release of restraints
- documenting your care.

Most facilities have a policy outlining the proper procedure for using restraints that conforms to TJC standards and the Centers for Medicare & Medicaid Services (CMS) regulations. Make sure you know your facility's policy well.

The law recognizes the legitimate use of restraints for acute medical and surgical care as a measure to prevent patient injury. It also recognizes the use of restraints or seclusion to manage violent or self-destructive behavior that jeopardizes the immediate physical safety of the patient, a staff member, or others.

The laws, they are a-changing . . .

State and federal regulations combine the standards for the use of restraints in acute medical and surgical care and seclusion for behavior management

into a single standard. This new standard focuses on protecting patients
from harmful behaviors, regardless of the patient's location. All health care
facilities governed by the CMS must adhere to these regulations.

Putting restraints on abusing restraints

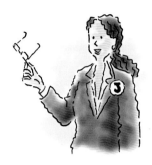

The law also states that a patient must be informed of patient's rights
upon admission to a health care facility. Specifically, a patient has
the right to be free from restraints or seclusion of any form imposed
by staff members as a means of coercion, discipline, convenience, or
retaliation. Restraints and seclusion may only be imposed to ensure
the immediate physical safety of the patient, staff members, or others
and must be discontinued at the earliest possible time.

Ordering restraints

A practitioner or other licensed independent practitioner (LIP) who is
responsible for the care of the patient and who is authorized to order
restraints or seclusion by hospital policy in accordance with state law
is allowed to order restraints for a patient. You may recommend to
the practitioner that physical restraints be ordered for a patient and
documentation your observations in the progress notes.

However, new regulations dictate that restraints or seclusion can
be used only when less restrictive interventions have been determined
to be ineffective to protect the patient or others from harm. Also, the
least restrictive type or technique of restraint or seclusion must be
used that will effectively protect the patient or others from harm.

Types of restraints

A *physical restraint* is any manual method or physical or mechanical
device, material, or equipment attached or adjacent to the patient's
body that the patient can't easily remove and that restricts freedom of
movement or normal access to the body. A *pharmaceutical restraint* is
a medication used as a restriction to manage the patient's behavior or
restrict the patient's freedom of movement that isn't part of standard
treatment for the patient's condition.

The earlier, the better

When restraints are used to ensure the safety of a nonviolent, non-
self-destructive patient, the order may be renewed as authorized by
the facility's policy. However, regardless of the length of the order,
restraints and seclusion must be discontinued at the earliest possible
time. (See *Physical restraint order*, page 150.)

Violent and self-destructive patients

When restraints or seclusion are used to manage violent or self-
destructive behavior that jeopardizes the immediate physical safety
of the patient, a staff member, or others, the patient must be seen
and evaluated face to face within 1 hour after initiating the restraint.

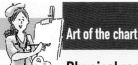

Art of the chart

Physical restraint order

A form and/or electronic physician order must be in the patient's chart before physical restraints are applied.

Date: _3/5/2017_   Time: _0315_

Reason for restraint use (circle all that apply):
1. Risk for self-harm
2. Risk for harm to others
3. High potential for removing tubes, equipment, or invasive lines
   ®subclavian CV line
4. Risk for causing significant disruption of the treatment environment
5. Other _____

Duration of restraint (Not to exceed 24 hr): _____ 24 hr

Type of restraint (circle all that apply):
Vest
Left mitt   Right mitt
Left wrist   Right wrist
Left ankle   Right ankle
Other _____

Practitioner's signature _____ J. Donnelly, MD

A trained registered nurse or physician's assistant may perform this assessment, but the practitioner or other LIP treating that patient must be consulted as soon as possible to further evaluate the patient's immediate status, response to the use of restraints, medical and behavioral history, and the need to continue or stop the restraint or seclusion.

One day at a time—no more

The restraint or seclusion order may be renewed up to a total of 24 hours, with different durations depending on age. The order may be renewed every 4 hours for adults 18 years and older, every 2 hours for children and adolescents between the ages of 9 and 17 years, and every hour for children younger than 9 years of age. After 24 hours, the practitioner or LIP must see and assess the patient before a new order is written.

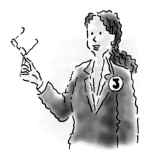

Getting into training

New regulations call for staff members who work with patients requiring restraints or seclusion to receive orientation training and annual staff retraining, according to facility policy. Staff members must demonstrate competency in applying and removing restraints and implementing seclusion as well as monitoring, assessing, and providing care for a patient in restraints or seclusion.

Hazard #7: Patients who request to see their charts

A patient has a legal right to read the medical record. The patient may ask to see it because of confusion related to the care being provided. First, ask the patient if there are questions regarding treatment and try to clear up any confusion.

If the patient still wants to see the record, check your facility's policy to see whether you or a hospital representative is required to be present while the patient reads the record. Document questions the patient asks about the record or any statements made about it by you or by the patient.

Don't just hand it over

Never release medical records to unauthorized people, including family members and police officers. Refer all requests from insurance companies to the appropriate administrator, and refer other requests to your nurse-manager. Be sure to notify your nurse-manager if you have any doubts about the validity of a request. The facility's administrator may also need to be notified.

Hazard #8: Patients who leave AMA

The law states that a mentally competent patient can leave a facility at any time. Having the patient sign an AMA form protects you, the practitioners, and the facility if problems arise from the unapproved discharge. However, even if the patient decides to leave AMA, you should attempt to provide discharge instructions related to care, such as wound care, if possible. Also, an attempt should be made to make sure that the patient has safe transportation from the facility.

Taking aim at the AMA form

The AMA form should clearly document that the patient:

- is leaving AMA
- has been advised of and understands the risks of leaving
- knows returning to the facility is permitted.

Use the patient's own words to describe the refusal. Here's what to include on the AMA form:

- names of relatives or friends notified of the patient's decision and the dates and times of the notifications
- explanation of the risks and consequences of the AMA discharge, as told to the patient, and the name of the person who provided the explanation

- discharge instructions or teaching provided
- other places the patient can go for follow-up care
- names of people accompanying the patient at discharge and the instructions given to them
- patient's mode of transportation and destination after discharge, if known.

If the patient leaves without anyone's knowledge or if refuses to sign the AMA form, check your facility's policy; you most likely will need to fill out an incident report in either situation.

Relate the patient's state

In the patient's medical record, document statements and actions that reflect the patient's mental state at the time the patient left your facility. Doing so helps protect you, the practitioner, security personnel, and the facility against a charge of negligence if the patient later claims that mental incompetence at the time of discharge and was improper supervision while in that state. (See *Leaving against medical advice.*)

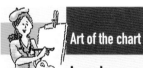

Art of the chart

Leaving against medical advice

When a patient leaves against medical advice (AMA), document it in the progress notes as shown below.

3/5/2017	1300	Pt found in room dressed in own clothes. Pt stated "I don't want any more tests or procedures. I'm going home." Explained to patient the risks of leaving the hospital, including the possibility of infection and unstable blood pressure. Pt stated "I understand—but I am leaving anyway. Just bring me the forms to sign out." Pt's son (Joe) in room but did not assist with convincing the pt to stay.————————— T. Vinson, RN
3/5/2017	1310	Notified Dr. J. McCarthy regarding pt's wish to sign out AMA. Agreed to see the patient ————————————————————— T. Vinson, RN
3/5/2017	1315	Dr. J. McCarthy in to see pt and discussed benefits of staying and risks of leaving. Pt still insists on leaving. Appt made with Dr. McCarthy's office. ————————————————————————————— T. Vinson, RN
3/5/2017	1330	Discharge instructions provided. Pt taken to son's car via wheelchair.—— ————————————————————————————— T. Vinson, RN

The case of the missing patient

Suppose a patient never says anything about leaving but, on rounds, you discover the patient is missing? If you can't find the patient in the facility, notify your nurse-manager (who should notify risk management), facility security, nursing supervisor, and the practitioner and then try to contact the patient's home. If the patient isn't there, call the police if you think the patient might perform self-harm or harm to others or if the patient left the hospital with any medical devices in place, such as an I.V. catheter.

Chart the time you discovered the patient missing, your attempts to find the patient, the people you notified, and other pertinent information.

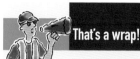

That's a wrap!

Legal pitfalls review

Basics
* Complete, accurate documentation proves that you're providing quality care and meeting standards.
* Faulty documentation is a pivotal issue in many malpractice cases.

Legal standards
* Nurse practice acts—state laws that designate nursing scope of practice
* American Nurses Association (ANA) requirements—standards set by the nursing profession
* Malpractice litigation—previous rulings, which are influenced by breach of duty, damage, and causation
* Facility policies and procedures—rules that are developed by each facility to identify standards of care

Defensive documentation
How to document
* Stick to facts.
* Avoid labeling.
* Be specific.
* Use neutral language.
* Eliminate bias.
* Keep the medical record intact.

What to document
* Significant situations
* Complete assessment data and care plan
* Discharge instructions

Other documentation tips
* Always document care when it's performed or shortly after.
* Never delegate your documentation.

Risk management and quality management goals
* Decreasing claims
* Reducing preventable accidents
* Controlling costs related to claims

Eight legal hazards
* Incident reports
* Informed consent
* Advance directives
* Patients who refuse treatment
* Documentation for unlicensed personnel
* Restraints
* Patients who request to see their medical record
* Patients who leave against medical advice

Suggested references

Bokar, V., and Perry, D.G. "Different Roles, Same Goal: Risk and Quality Management Partnering for Patient Safety. By the ASHRM Monographs Task Force," *Journal of Healthcare Risk Management* 27(2):17-23, 2007.

Chesanow, C. "Malpractice: When to Settle a Suit and When to Fight," 2013. Available: https://www.medscape.com/viewarticle/811323.

Ferrell, K.G. "Documentation, Part 2: The Best Evidence of Care. Complete and Accurate Charting can be Crucial to Exonerating Nurses in Civil Lawsuits," *The American Journal of Nursing* 107(7):61-64, July 2007.

Lockwood, W. "Documentation: Accurate and Legal," 2017. Available: http://www .rn.org/courses/coursematerial-66.pdf.

Meldi, D., et al. "The Big Three: A Side by Side Matrix Comparing Hospital Accrediting Agencies," 2009. Available: https://www.hfap.org/mediacenter /NAMSS%20Synergy%20JanFeb09_Accreditation%20Grid.pdf.

Rosenberg, S. "How to Avoid Getting Sued," 2017. Available: https://www.medscape .com/viewarticle/880454.

Russell, K.A. "Nurse Practice Acts Guide and Govern Nursing Practice," *Journal of Nurse Regulation* 3(3):36-42, 2012. Available: https://www.ncsbn.org/2012_JNR _NPA_Guide.pdf.

US Legal, Inc. "Medical Malpractice Law and Legal Definition," 2016. Available: https://definitions.uslegal.com/m/medical-malpractice/.

US Legal, Inc. "Nursing Law and Legal Definition," 2016. Available: https://definitions .uslegal.com/n/nursing/.

Chapter 7

Documenting procedures

Just the facts

In this chapter, you'll learn:

♦ documentation requirements for several common nursing procedures

♦ guidelines for documenting medication administration and intravenous (I.V.) therapy

♦ documentation guidelines for assisted and miscellaneous procedures.

Guidelines for documenting procedures

Your notes about routine nursing procedures usually appear in the patient's chart, on flow sheets, or on graphic forms. Whatever your health care facility's requirements are, you must include this information in your documentation:

- what procedure was performed
- when it was performed
- who performed it
- how it was performed
- how well the patient tolerated it
- adverse reactions to the procedure, if any
- interventions provided related to the adverse reactions and the patient's response to those interventions.

The sections that follow outline information that must be documented for several nursing procedures.

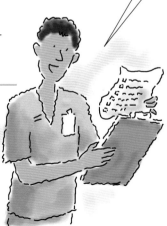

Take the time to document accurately, objectively, thoroughly, consistently, and legibly—in routine and exceptional situations.

Medication administration

A medication administration record (MAR) is part of most documentation systems. Medication administration may be documented electronically (called eMAR), often using bar code technology, or on paper with the use of a medication Kardex. In either case, it's the central record of medication orders and their execution and is part of the patient's permanent record.

You document MARvelously

When administering and documenting medications, follow these guidelines:

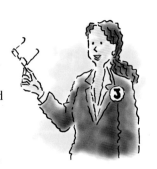

- Follow your facility's policies and procedures for verifying medication orders and administration.
- Verify that the right patient's name appears on the eMAR, or record or label each page of a paper MAR with the patient's full name, medical record number, and allergy information.
- If transcribing a medication order, *use only standard abbreviations. Remember that The Joint Commission prohibits the use of certain abbreviations (those that appear on the "Do Not Use" list).* Electronic order entries are set up to also follow the "Do Not Use" rules.
- Before administering any medication, confirm the patient's identity using at least two patient identifiers.
- Avoid distractions and interruptions when preparing and administering medication to prevent medication errors.
- Compare the medication label to the order in the patient's medical record.
- Check the patient's medical record for an allergy or contraindication to the prescribed medication. If an allergy or contraindications exist, don't administer the medication and notify the practitioner.
- Check the expiration date on the medication. If the medication is expired, return it to the pharmacy and obtain new medication.
- Visually inspect the solution for particles or discoloration or other loss of integrity; don't administer the medication if integrity is compromised.
- Discuss any unresolved concerns about the medication with the patient's practitioner.
- If the patient is receiving the medication for the first time, teach the patient and family (if appropriate) about potential adverse reactions or other concerns related to the medication.
- Verify that the medication is being administered at the proper time, in the prescribed dose, and by the correct route to reduce the risk for medication errors.
- If your facility uses barcode technology, scan your identification badge, the patient's identification bracelet, and the medication's barcode.
- If a medication requires an independent double-check with another nurse, complete this step before administration. If there are no discrepancies, administer the medication. If discrepancies exist, rectify them before beginning administering the medication.
- If using a medication Kardex, after administering the medication, sign your full name, licensure status, and initials in the appropriate spaces.

- Document medication administration immediately after each dose is administered so that another nurse doesn't inadvertently repeat the dose.
- If a specific assessment parameter must be monitored before administration of a drug, document this requirement. For example, when digoxin is administered, the patient's pulse rate must be monitored and documented.
- If you didn't give a medication, follow the procedure for documenting this omission per the eMAR system used. If using a medication Kardex, circle the time and document the reason for the omission.
- Record any adverse reactions to the prescribed medication, the date and time the practitioner was notified, prescribed interventions, and the patient's response to those interventions.

As needed medications

Document all as needed (p.r.n.) drugs when administered, including the reason for giving the drug and the patient's response. For specific drugs given p.r.n., follow these guidelines:

- For eye, ear, or nose drops, document the number of drops administered as well as the administration route.
- For suppositories, document the type (rectal, vaginal, or urethral) and how the patient tolerated it.
- For dermal medications, document the location of the area where you applied the medication and the condition of the skin or wound.
- For dermal patches, chart the location of the patch.
- For intravenous (I.V.), intramuscular (I.M.), or subcutaneous medications, document the location of administration.

No room for exceptions

If you administer p.r.n. drugs according to accepted standards, you don't need to document more specific information, unless an unusual event occurs.

Drug abuse or refusal

If the patient refuses or abuses medications, describe the event in the patient's medical record. The eMAR system may have specific methods for documenting this event. Here are some situations that require careful documentation:

- You discover nonprescribed drugs at the patient's bedside. Document the type of medication (pill or powder), the amount of medication, and its color and shape. (You may wish to send the drug to the pharmacy for identification.) Follow your facility's policy regarding the completion of the appropriate report.

- You found a supply of prescribed drugs in the patient's bedside table, indicating that the patient is not taking the medications administered. Record the type and amount of medication. Report this situation to the nurse-manager because education may need to be provided to nursing staff regarding proper medication administration.
- You notice a sudden change in the patient's behavior after visitors left the room and you suspect them of giving the patient opioids or other drugs. Document how the patient appeared before the visitors came and afterward. Notify the practitioner immediately and follow your facility's policy. Complete the incident report, if applicable.
- You offer prescribed medications and the patient refuses to take them. Document the refusal, the reason for it (if the patient tells you), and the medication. This prevents the refusal from being misinterpreted as an omission or a medication error on your part.
- You held medication related to parameters that the practitioners ordered or established protocol (such as a heart rate less than 60 beats/minute for administering digoxin) or due to the patient's condition (such as vomiting). Document the reason for holding the medication and the date and time the practitioner was notified and any orders the practitioner provided (such as changing the medication to I.V.).

Paging the practitioner . . .

Report any medication abuse or refusal to the practitioner. When you do so, document the name of the practitioner, the response, and the date and time of notification.

Controlled substance administration

Whenever you give a controlled substance, such as a narcotic, you must document it according to federal, state, and facility regulations. These regulations require you to:
- remove the drug from the dispensing unit, following the units prompt for drug count or cosignature or sign out the drug on the appropriate form
- verify that the drug dose is correct before administering it
- have another nurse witness and document if you must waste part of a narcotic dose.

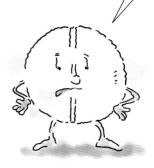

Document controlled substance administration according to federal, state, and facility regulations.

Double team

Depending on your facility's policy, two nurses should be present to count controlled substances each shift—preferably an oncoming and off-going nurse. If you discover a discrepancy in the controlled substance count that cannot be resolved immediately, report it, following your facility's policy. Also, file an incident report. An investigation will follow, per facility policy.

I.V. therapy

More than 80% of hospitalized patients receive some form of I.V. therapy, such as fluid or electrolyte replacement, total parenteral nutrition (TPN), medication infusions, and blood products. Document all facets of I.V. therapy carefully, including subsequent complications.

Basic documentation

After establishing an I.V. route, document:
- date, time, and venipuncture site
- equipment used such as the type and gauge of the catheter
- number of venipuncture attempts made, the type of assistance required (if applicable), and the patient's response
- any adverse events, such as a hematoma, interventions provided, and the patients response to those interventions.

Once per shift (or according to your facility's or unit's policy), document:
- type, amount, and flow rate of I.V. fluid
- condition of the I.V. site
- that you flushed the I.V. catheter and what medication or solution you used.

Note: Most facilities require documentation of I.V. fluids or flush in the MAR.

Document each time you change the insertion site, venipuncture device, or I.V. tubing. Also, document the reason you changed the I.V. site, such as extravasation, phlebitis, occlusion, patient removal, or a routine change. Document discontinuation of an I.V. and that the catheter was intact when removed.

Getting complicated

Document complications precisely. For example, record if extravasation occurs and what interventions you took, such as stopping the I.V. infusion, assessing the amount of fluid infiltrated, and notifying the practitioner.

If a chemotherapeutic drug extravasates, stop the I.V. infusion immediately and follow the procedure specified by your health care facility. Document the appearance of the I.V. site, the treatment you gave (especially antidotes), and the kind of dressing you applied. Document the amount of any discarded medication.

If the patient has an allergic reaction during I.V. therapy, stop the infusion and notify the practitioner immediately. Then document all pertinent information about the reaction as well as your interventions and the patient's response.

Don't forget the family

Record patient and family teaching, such as explaining the purpose of I.V. therapy, describing the procedure itself, and discussing possible complications. Document their understanding of the teaching provided and if follow-up teaching is needed.

TPN

If a patient is receiving TPN, document:
- type and location of the central venous access device (CVAD)
- condition of the insertion site and type of dressing as well as when it was last changed
- verification of the components of the infusion bags with the practitioner's order using a double-check system with another nurse
- volume and rate of the solution infused.

We interrupt this service . . .

When you discontinue a central I.V. catheter for TPN, record:
- date and time
- type of dressing applied
- appearance of the administration site
- why it was discontinued—for example, a practitioner's order, infiltration, or phlebitis.

Blood transfusions

Whenever you administer blood or blood components—such as whole blood, packed red blood cells, plasma, platelets, or cryoprecipitates—use proper identification and crossmatching procedures.
- patient's name
- patient's medical record number
- patient's blood group or type
- patient's and donor's rhesus (Rh) factor
- crossmatch data
- blood bank identification number
- expiration date of the product

The Joint Commission states that blood or blood component must be identified by two licensed health care professionals, both of whom sign the slip that comes with the blood and verify that the information is correct, unless using automated identification technology, which only requires a one-person verification process.

After you determine that the information on the blood bag label is correct or an automated scanning system verifies the correct patient and blood component, you may administer the transfusion. Documentation on the transfusion administration record should include:
- dates and times the transfusion was started and completed
- names of the health care professionals who verified the information

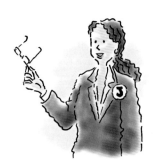

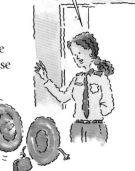

I'm sorry but I'm going to need to see six forms of identification please.

- type and gauge of the I.V. catheter
- total amount of the transfusion and normal saline solution infused
- patient's vital signs before the transfusion, 15 minutes after the transfusion is started, and after the transfusion is completed, according to your facility's policy
- infusion device used, if any, and its flow rate
- blood warming unit used, if any
- patient's response to the transfusion.

Accounting for autotransfusions

If the patient receives autologous blood, document the amount retrieved and reinfused in the intake and output (I&O) records. Document laboratory tests during and after the autotransfusion, paying special attention to the coagulation profile, hematocrit, and arterial blood gas (ABG), hemoglobin, and calcium levels. Also document the patient's pretransfusion, midtransfusion, and posttransfusion vital signs.

Reacting to a suspected transfusion reaction

If the patient develops a suspected transfusion reaction, stop the transfusion immediately, hang new tubing with normal saline solution running, and notify the practitioner. Documentation of the event should include:
- time and date of the reaction
- type and amount of infused blood or blood products
- times you started and stopped the transfusion
- clinical signs in the order of occurrence
- patient's vital signs per facility protocol
- urine specimens and blood samples sent to the laboratory for analysis
- date, time, and name of the practitioner notified, orders received, interventions provided, and the patient's response to those interventions.

You will need to send any noninfused blood and tubing back to the blood bank. Follow your facility's policy. Document the suspected transfusion reaction in the transfusion administration record in the electronic health record (EHR), if available. If not using an electronic system, write a nurses' note describing the event. (See *Suspected transfusion reaction*, page 162.)

Surgical incision care

When a patient returns from surgery, obtain and document vital signs according to facility policy and level of consciousness (LOC) and carefully record information about the surgical incision, drains, and the care you provide.

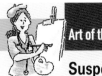

Art of the chart

Suspected transfusion reaction

Here is an example of how to document a suspected transfusion reaction.

1/16/2017	1130	Pt c/o nausea and chills. Transfusion of PRBC's initiated at 1100 with
		approximately 100 mL infused. Transfusion discontinued and NSS solution
		started with new tub ing at 100 ml/hr. VS: Temp 99.4, BP Call placed to
		Dr. J. Dunn. Per policy and procedure, blood bank notified and bag of PRBC's
		returned to lab. ———————————————————— A. Grasso, RN
1/16/2017	1145	Dr. J. Dunn notified of pt's condition. Pt given diphenhydramine 50 mg I.V.
		and I.V. of NSS to continue at 100 ml/hr. Urine specimen obtained and sent
		to lab. Lab technician in and obtained specimens per policy and procedure.
		Pt no longer nauseated or c/o chills. VS: Temp 99, BP 164/86, HR 100,
		RR 24. Pox 96% ————————————————————— A. Grasso, RN

If your EHR has specific screens designated for postoperative evaluation, be sure to utilize them correctly. If not using an EHR, complete a nurses' note describing the patient's postop condition on arrival from the postanesthesia care unit (PACU). (See *Postop observations*.)

Records that get around

Study the records that travel with the patient from the PACU. (See *Roaming records*, page 163.)

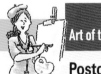

Art of the chart

Postop observations

Here is an example of an initial postoperative note after the patient arrives to an assigned room.

1/17/2017	1030	Pt received from PACU into rm 1410. Bedside report received from
		C. Harris RN. Pt alert and oriented x4. Pain level "1" on scale 0 to 10.
		Dressing on abdomen intact with small (2 cm) area of serous drain age noted
		and marked. #18g I.V. intact in LH. Lactated Ringers solution infusing at
		75 ml/hr. Site without redness or edema. Skin warm and dry. Respirations
		nonlabored. Sequential therapy stockings in place and functioning. See VS sheet.
		Oriented to room. Call bell within reach and bed in low position. ——— D. Lin, RN

Roaming records

When your patient recovers from anesthesia and is transferred from the postanesthesia care unit (PACU) to the patient's assigned room for ongoing recovery and care, as the nurse, you're responsible for the documents that travel with the patient and are part of the medical record. Some information may be documented electronically, with other information documented on specific flow sheets. Make sure that all flow sheets contain the patient's information, including the patient's name, date of birth, medical record number, account number, and date of admission.

Part 1: Preanesthesia record
The preanesthesia record should include information about the care provided before the surgical procedure started. It should include:
- allergy information
- vital signs and a cardiac rhythm strip
- the date and time that the patient last ingested food or water
- the site of intravenous (I.V.) insertions (and catheter gauge)
- any medications administered and the time of administration
- pain level
- removal of dentures, contacts, glasses, or hearing aids
- preparation of the surgical site (such as clipping and scrubbing)
- application of venous thromboembolism devices, such as compression stockings or sequential compression therapy.

Any patient teaching should also be documented, including the patient's understanding of the teaching provided.

Part 2: Operation
The operative section describes the surgery performed and should include:
- the exact procedure performed
- the type and dosage of anesthetics
- how long the patient was anesthetized
- the patient's vital signs throughout surgery
- the volume of fluid, including blood, lost and replaced
- drugs administered, with administration times noted
- surgical complications and interventions provided, along with the patient's response
- tourniquet time
- drains, tubes, implants, or dressings used during surgery and removed or still in place.

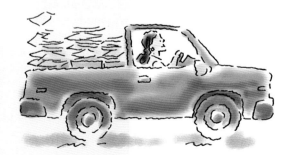

(continued)

Roaming records *(continued)*

Part 3: Postanesthesia period

The postanesthesia part of the record includes information about:

• vital signs, including temperature and pulse oximetry

• level of consciousness (LOC)

• pain medications and pain control devices the patient received and how the patient responded to them

• surgical incision dressings or site, if open to air

• interventions that should continue on the unit, such as frequent circulatory, motor, and neurologic checks if the patient underwent leg surgery and had a tourniquet on for a long time

• the patient's postanesthesia recovery scores on arrival and discharge in the areas of activity level, respiration, circulation, and LOC

• unusual events or complications that occurred in the PACU; for example, nausea or vomiting, shivering, hypothermia, arrhythmias, central anticholinergic syndrome, sore throat, back or neck pain, corneal abrasion, tooth loss during intubation, swollen lips or tongue, pharyngeal or laryngeal abrasion, and postspinal headache as well as any interventions provided for these events and the patient's response to those interventions

• time of transfer (or discharge) and the room the patient was moved to.

Who's up first?

Look for a practitioner's order stating when the first dressing change should occur and who should perform that dressing change. If you'll be performing it, document:

• type of wound care performed (sterile or clean technique)

• wound's appearance (size, color, condition of margins, type of sutures [or absence of sutures], and presence of necrotic tissue); odor, if any; location of drains; and drainage characteristics (type, color, consistency, and amount)

• condition of skin around drain or wound

• type and amount of dressing

• additional wound care procedures, such as drain management, irrigation, packing, or application of a topical medication

• how the patient tolerated the dressing change

• teaching provided to the patient (or family, if applicable), understanding of the teaching, and if additional teaching is needed.

Detailed care and discharge data

Document special or detailed wound care instructions and pain management measures on the nursing care plan. Also, chart the color and amount of measurable drainage on the I&O form.

If the patient needs wound care after discharge, provide patient teaching to include patient and family members, if present, and document it. Chart that you explained aseptic technique, described how to examine the wound for infection or other complications, demonstrated how to change the dressing, and gave written instructions for home care. Optimally, have the patient or family demonstrate changing the dressing and document if care was performed correctly. Include the patient's understanding of the instructions, and document if the patient or family can perform wound care measures or if further teaching is needed.

Pacemaker care

If the patient has a transvenous or permanent pacemaker inserted, record:
- date and time of placement
- name of the practitioner who inserted the pacemaker (transvenous), if performed at the bedside
- reason for placement
- pacemaker settings and type
- patient's response to the procedure
- patient's LOC and vital signs, including which arm you used to obtain the blood pressure reading
- complications, such as chest pain and signs of infection
- interventions such as X-rays to verify correct electrode placement
- medications that may have been given before or during the procedure.

Obtain a rhythm strip prior to insertion, after insertion, and every 4 hours and make sure it includes the patient's name and the date and time.

If the patient has a transcutaneous pacemaker, document the reason for pacing, the time pacing started, the pacemaker settings, and the locations of the electrodes. Be sure to obtain rhythm strips and post in the patient's chart. Also document the patient's tolerance of the procedure, any sedation or pain medication administered, and the effectiveness of interventions. If the transcutaneous pacemaker is ordered as "standby," be sure to note that it is available at the patient's bedside and that pacing pads are in place.

If your EHR has specific screens designated for pacemaker documentation, be sure to utilize them correctly. If not using an EHR, complete a nurses' note describing the procedure, including the patient's condition.

Peritoneal dialysis

If your patient is receiving peritoneal dialysis, monitor and document the patient's response to treatment during and after the procedure.
Be sure to document:

- patient's vital signs per facility protocol
- abrupt changes in the patient's condition and the date and time that you notified the practitioner, any interventions ordered and performed, and the patient's response to those interventions
- type of peritoneal dialysis being performed (continuous ambulatory peritoneal dialysis [CAPD] or continuous cycling peritoneal dialysis [CCPD])
- amount and type of dialysate infused and drained and medications added
- effluent's characteristics (color, clarity, and odor) and the assessed negative or positive fluid balance at the end of each infusion-dwell-drain cycle
- patient's daily weight (immediately after the drain phase) and abdominal girth when the treatment ends; note the time of day and the weighing and measuring technique.
- physical assessment findings, including the condition of the patient's skin at the dialysis catheter site
- fluid status
- equipment problems, such as kinked tubing or mechanical malfunction and your interventions
- patient's reports of unusual discomfort or pain and your interventions
- any break in aseptic technique and the date and time that you notified the practitioner
- whether the patient, family member, or dialysis technician performs the peritoneal dialysis procedure.

If your EHR has specific screens designated for dialysis documentation, be sure to utilize them correctly. If not using an EHR, complete a nurses' note describing the procedure and the patient's condition. (See *Peritoneal dialysis documentation*, page 167.)

Peritoneal lavage

For the patient experiencing peritoneal lavage, document:

- patient's vital signs before, during, and after the procedure
- name of the practitioner performing the procedure
- condition of the incision site
- type and size of the peritoneal catheter used
- type and amount of solution instilled into the peritoneal cavity
- amount and color of the fluid withdrawn from the peritoneal cavity and whether it flowed freely in and out

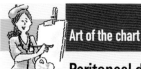

Art of the chart

Peritoneal dialysis documentation

2/20/2017	0900	Pt receiving CAPD via midabdominal peritoneal catheter. Catheter site without redness, edema, or tenderness. Therapy initiated using 4.25 dialysate with 500 units of heparin and 2 mEq KCl. 1,500 ml infused and catheter clamped. Dwell time: 4 hours. Pt weight: 110 kg. Pt teaching provided regarding procedure. Pt states understanding. ———————— A. Taylor, RN
2/20/2017	1300	CAPD set to drain via gravity. ———————————— A. Taylor, RN
2/20/2017	1330	CAPD drainage complete. 1,650 ml returned. Drainage clear. Pale yellow. Pt tolerated procedure. Pt weight: 108 kg. ——————— A. Taylor, RN

- what specimens were obtained and sent to the laboratory for analysis
- complications that occurred, such as symptoms of shock (tachycardia, decreased blood pressure, diaphoresis, dyspnea, and vertigo); the date, time, and name of the practitioner notified; any interventions provided; and the patient's response to those interventions
- patient teaching provided, the patient's understanding of that teaching, and if follow-up teaching is needed.

Chest tube

If your patient has a chest tube inserted, initially record:
- date and time of the insertion
- name of the practitioner who inserted the chest tube (if performed at the bedside)
- site of insertion
- type of dressing applied
- type of system used
- amount of suction applied (if any) to the pleural cavity
- presence or absence of bubbling or fluctuation in the water-seal chamber
- amount and type of drainage (if any)
- patient's respiratory status, including pulse oximetry and breath sounds

- chest X-ray obtained for verification
- patient teaching provided, understanding of that teaching, and if additional teaching is needed.

The documentation goes on and on

Ongoing documentation includes:

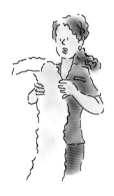

- color, consistency, and amount of thoracic drainage in the collection chamber as well as the time and date of each observation
- presence or absence of bubbling or fluctuation in the water-seal chamber
- patient's respiratory status, including pulse oximetry readings
- condition of the chest dressings
- dressing changes and the patient's skin condition at the chest tube site
- type, amount, and route of pain medication administered, and the effectiveness of treatment
- complications, such as cyanosis, rapid or shallow breathing, crepitus, chest pain, or excessive bleeding; the time and date you notified the practitioner; interventions you provided; and the patient's response to those interventions
- patient-teaching sessions and activities you taught the patient to perform, such as coughing and deep breathing exercises, sitting upright, and splinting the insertion site to minimize pain
- change or discontinuation of suction level and chest X-rays obtained
- removal of chest tube and patient response.

If your EHR has specific screens designated for chest tube use, be sure to utilize them correctly. If not using an EHR, complete a nurses' note describing the procedure and the patient's condition. (See Documenting a chest tube.)

Art of the chart

Documenting a chest tube

Here is an example of an assessment of a patient's chest tube.

2/22/2017	0800	R posterior chest tube intact to 20 cm of suction. Draining small amounts of serous fluid (20 ml last shift). No air leak noted. Dressing dry and intact. No drainage noted. No crepitus present. Lungs clear with diminished breath sounds on R side. Pt denies pain. Performed coughing and deep breathing exercises when asked. —————————— N. Sigfried, RN

Cardiac monitoring

Cardiac monitoring is usually a routine component of specific units, and application of the monitoring unit does not need to be documented. For the patient receiving cardiac monitoring, include in your documentation:

- rhythm strip readings per unit routine or with any rhythm change, labeled with the patient's name and the date and time
- alarm limits are set appropriately for the patient's current condition and that the alarms are turned on, functioning properly, and audible to staff
- date and time the practitioner notified of rhythm changes, interventions provided, and the patient's response to rhythm changes.

Keep on chartin'

If the patient is to continue cardiac monitoring after discharge, document:

- patient and family teaching regarding the reason for monitoring and how long it will be performed, event recording, and equipment care
- referrals to equipment suppliers, home health agencies, and other community resources.

Chest physiotherapy

Whenever you perform chest physiotherapy, document:

- date and time of your interventions
- patient's positions for secretion drainage and how long the patient remains in each
- chest segments you percussed or vibrated
- characteristics of the secretion expelled, including color, amount, odor, viscosity, and the presence of blood
- patient's tolerance of the chest physiotherapy
- breath sounds before and after treatment
- patient teaching regarding the procedure, the patient's understanding of that teaching, and if additional teaching is needed
- complications, name of the practitioner notified, interventions provided, and the patient's response to those interventions.

If your EHR has specific screens designated for chest physiotherapy, be sure to utilize them correctly. If not using an EHR, complete a nurses' note describing the procedure and the patient's condition. (See Performing chest physiotherapy, page 170.)

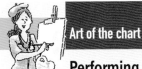

Art of the chart

Performing chest physiotherapy

2/28/2017	1130	Explained procedure to pt and answered all questions. Pt stated.
		understanding Lungs with crackles in the LUL. Pt placed in Trendelen
		burg position on R side. Chest percussion and vibration performed on
		L side of chest. Pt tolerated procedure and produced a moderate amount
		of thick yellow sputum. Lungs clear to auscultation. ——————— H. Moppert, RN

Mechanical ventilation

For patients receiving mechanical ventilation, initially document:
- date and time of endotracheal (ET) intubation with initial verification of placement (CO_2 detection, auscultation, chest movement)
- name of practitioner who inserted the ET tube
- any medication administered, including dose and site of administration
- size of ET tube and placement number of the proximal end of the ET tube at the lip level
- chest X-ray verification of placement
- use of continuous waveform capnography (if available)
- initial ventilator settings and time of ABG testing
- patient's responses to mechanical ventilation, including vital signs, breath sounds, use of accessory muscles, secretions, I&O, weight, and pulse oximetry readings.

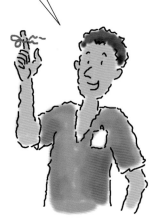

Don't forget to document the patient's responses to mechanical ventilation.

Take a deep breath—then document!

Throughout use of mechanical ventilation, document:
- ventilator settings every shift, any changes, and the patient's response to those changes
- results of ABG analyses and oxygen saturation findings
- position of the head of the bed to decrease ventilator-associated events
- sedation and pain medication administered, including holding sedation for spontaneous wakening trials and the patient's response
- duration of spontaneous breathing trials and the ability to participate in weaning

- interventions to increase mobility, protect skin integrity, or enhance ventilation; for example, active or passive range-of-motion exercises, turning or positioning the patient, and chest physiotherapy
- suctioning and the presence and characteristics of secretions obtained
- type and frequency of oral care provided
- assessment findings related to LOC, peripheral circulation, urine output, decreased cardiac output, fluid volume excess, or dehydration
- complications, name of the practitioner notified, interventions provided, and the patient's response to those interventions
- removal of the ET tube (per practitioner's order), the oxygen delivery device utilized (and the amount of oxygen delivered), and the patient's response, including ABG results and pulse oximetry readings
  Note: If the patient is accidently extubated, or the patient removes the ET tube, most facilities require an incident report be completed.
- patient and family teaching provided, their understanding of the teaching, and if follow-up teaching is needed
- patient and family teaching provided for the patient requiring ventilator support at home, including discussions and demonstrations related to ventilator use, suctioning, signs and symptoms of complications, and when to notify the practitioner
- referrals to equipment vendors, home health agencies, and other community resources.

The respiratory therapist is responsible for documentation of mechanical ventilation, along with the nurse.

If your EHR has specific screens designated for mechanical ventilation, be sure to utilize them correctly. If not using an EHR, complete a nurses' note describing the procedure and the patient's condition. (See Documenting mechanical ventilation.)

Art of the chart

Documenting mechanical ventilation

Here is an example of documentation of a patient being weaned from mechanical ventilation.

3/28/2017	1100	Pt placed on CPAP of 0 with O₂ at 40% for weaning. Pt alert and nods
		understanding of procedure. Lungs clear. No respiratory distress. RR 16.
		Pox: 95%. ABG scheduled for 1200. —————————————— J. Devine, RN
3/28/2017	1200	Pt tolerating T-piece. No signs of respiratory distress. RR: 18. Pox 96%. ABG
		obtained from L radial artery by RT. ———————————— J. Devine, RN

Nasogastric tube insertion, use, and removal

A nasogastric (NG) tube may be inserted for decompression or empty-ing of the stomach or to administer medications or enteral feeding. After you insert an NG tube, document:

- patient teaching provided regarding the reason for the NG tube and the insertion procedure
- type and size of the NG tube
- date, time, insertion route, and reason for insertion
- type and amount of suction (if any)
- amount, color, consistency, and odor of the fluid aspirated
- how the patient tolerated the procedure
- method of placement verification (e.g., testing the pH of the gastric aspirate or X-ray), which should be performed on insertion, at regular intervals, (per facility policy and procedure) and before medication administration.

Using the NG tube

Ongoing documentation of the use of an NG tube should include:

- regular verification of placement per facility policy and procedure
- amount and type of drainage, if connected to suction device
- if used to administer enteral feedings: type and amount of feeding administered, with documentation of tube placement before ini-tiation and the patient's tolerance of the tube feeding provided
- signs and symptoms of complications, such as nausea, vomiting, and abdominal distention; name of the practitioner notified; inter-ventions provided; and the patient's response to those interventions. Record input and output information about irrigations, medica-tion instillations, feedings, and drainage.

If your EHR has specific screens designated for NG tube use, be sure to utilize them correctly. If not using an EHR, complete a nurses' note describing the procedure and the patient's condition. (See Documentation of nasogastric tube insertion, page 173.)

The tube is removed—so document some more!

After you remove an NG tube, document:

- date and time of removal
- how the patient tolerated the procedure
- unusual events accompanying tube removal, such as nausea, vom-iting, abdominal distention, and food intolerance; interventions provided; and the patient's response to those interventions
- gastrointestinal (GI) assessment, including bowel sounds and type and amount of bowel movements.

Art of the chart

Documentation of nasogastric tube insertion

Here is an example of documenting the insertion of a nasogastric (NG) tube.

1/30/2017	2100	Pt with continuous vomiting. NG tube to intermittent suction ordered by
		Dr. Bolding. Explained procedure to patient and family regarding need for
		NG and the procedure. Pt states understanding. #12 Fr NG tube inserted
		via R nostril and secured to nose. Aspirated 350 ml bile-colored fluid.
		X-ray ordered for verification of placement. Pt tolerated procedure. NG
		tube clamped at present. ———————————————— D. Harris, RN

Seizure occurrence and management

If your patient has a seizure while hospitalized, document:
- date and time the seizure began and its duration
- precipitating factors, including auralike sensations reported by the patient
- involuntary behavior occurring before the seizure, such as lip smacking, chewing movements, or hand and eye movements; behavior occurring during the seizure, such as tonic–clonic movements, and postictal behavior
- incontinence, vomiting, or salivation during the seizure
- patient's vital signs during (if possible) and after the seizure
- your assessment of the patient's postseizure mental and physical status
- what and when you reported to the practitioner, interventions provided (including medications), and the patient's response to those interventions
- what seizure precautions were initiated.

If your EHR has specific screens designated for seizure documentation (which may be part of the neurologic assessment screens), be sure to utilize them correctly. If not using an EHR, complete a nurses' note describing the event and the patient's condition. (See Seizure documentation, page 174.)

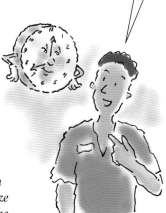

Document the date and time the patient's seizure began and its duration.

Suture and staple removal

If the practitioner writes an order for you to remove sutures or staples, document:
- date and time the sutures were removed and the patient's response
- appearance of the suture line

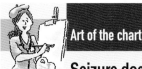

Art of the chart

Seizure documentation

Here is an example of documentation after the patient experiences a seizure.

4/30/2017	1615	Pt observed having tonic—clonic seizure movements in bed lasting 3 minutes.
		Pt in continent of urine during seizure. Safety measures provided during
		seizure (head and airway protection). Seizure pads present on side rails.
		Pt placed on L side. Presently lethargic. VS: BP 130/90, HR 110, RR 14, Pox
		94%. Call placed to Dr. Defabio. ——————————————— B. Chao, RN

- appearance of the wound site, including the presence of purulent drainage
- if and when you notified the practitioner for any issues, interventions provided, and the patient's response to those interventions
- if and when you collected a wound specimen and sent it to the laboratory for analysis
- patient teaching provided, understanding of that teaching, and if additional teaching is needed.

    If your EHR has specific screens designated for suture removal, be sure to utilize them correctly. If not using an EHR, complete a nurses' note describing the procedure and the patient's condition.

Tube feedings

When documenting your care of a patient receiving tube feedings, document:

- the kind of tube feeding the patient is receiving (such as duodenal or jejunal feedings or a continuous drip or bolus)
- amount, rate, route, and method of feeding (with continuous feedings, document the hourly rate)
- where the tube feeding is being administered, such as via NG tube, enteral tube, or percutaneous endoscopic gastrostomy (PEG) tube
- GI assessment, including bowel sounds, abdominal pain, and type and amount of bowel movements
- patient's tolerance of the feeding, complications, and your interventions
- dilution strength if you need to dilute the formula (e.g., half-strength or three-quarters strength)
- time, amount, and type of flush solution, if applicable

- replacement of the tube and how the patient tolerated the procedure, if applicable
- amount of gastric residual, if applicable, and if tube feeding was held
- laboratory results, such as urine and serum glucose, serum electrolyte, and blood urea nitrogen levels as well as serum osmolality values
- feeding complications, such as hyperglycemia, glycosuria, and diarrhea; the time you notified the practitioner; interventions provided; and the patient's response to those interventions
- patient and family teaching provided, their understanding of that teaching, and if follow-up teaching is needed. Provide additional teaching, with return demonstration, if the patient will continue receiving tube feedings after discharge.
- referrals to suppliers or support agencies.

If your EHR has specific screens designated for tube feeding administration, be sure to utilize them correctly. Also document in the I&O screens. If not using an EHR, complete a nurses' note describing the procedure and the patient's condition and document I&O appropriately.

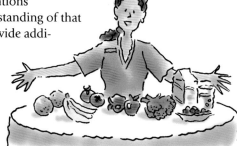

When giving tube feedings, be sure to document the patient's tolerance of the feeding formula.

Obtaining an arterial blood sample

When you obtain blood for ABG analysis, document:
- patient's vital signs and temperature
- results of Allen's test
- arterial puncture site
- indications of circulatory impairment, such as swelling, discoloration, pain, numbness, or tingling in the bandaged arm or leg, and bleeding at the puncture site
- date and time you drew the blood sample or name of the person drawing the sample
- how long you applied pressure to the site to control bleeding
- type and amount of oxygen therapy that the patient was receiving (if applicable).

If your EHR has specific screens designated for ABG testing, which may be part of the respiratory assessment screens, be sure to utilize them correctly. If not using an EHR, complete a nurses' note describing the procedure and the patient's condition.

Need an ABG analysis? That's another form!

When filling out a laboratory request form for ABG analysis, include:
- patient's current temperature
- oxygen concentration via device or fraction of inspired oxygen and tidal volume if receiving mechanical ventilation.

Documenting assisted procedures

When you assist a practitioner during a procedure, you have the added responsibilities of providing patient support and teaching, evaluating the patient's response, and carefully documenting the procedure.

Procedures may change, but the documentation remains the same

Regardless of the procedure, confirm that an informed consent was signed, if applicable. Additionally, you must always document:

- date, time, and name of the procedure
- practitioner who performed it and assistants involved
- the time-out conducted before the procedure started (if indicated), including who was involved in the time-out and the confirmation of the right patient, right site, procedure and, as applicable, all relevant information and necessary equipment were available
- how it was performed
- medications administered, including the medication strength, dose, route of administration, and date and time of administration (which may be completed using the eMAR system)
- how the patient tolerated the procedure
- complications or adverse reactions to the procedure, if any, interventions provided, and the patient's response to those interventions
- any teaching provided to the patient and family, their understanding of that teaching, and if follow-up teaching is needed.

The section that follows describes documentation for several procedures during which you may assist the practitioner.

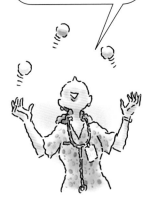

While assisting a practitioner during a procedure, I have another important job to do—document the procedure. That's a lot of responsibilities to juggle!

Bone marrow aspiration

After assisting the practitioner with bone marrow aspiration, document:

- date and time of the procedure
- name of the practitioner performing the procedure
- medication administered, including the medication strength, dose, route of administration, and date and time of administration
- the time-out conducted before the procedure started, including who was involved in the time-out, and the confirmation of the right patient, right site, procedure and, as applicable, all relevant information and necessary equipment were available
- location and appearance of the aspiration site, including bleeding and drainage
- patient's vital signs before and after the procedure
- how the patient tolerated the procedure
- complications or adverse reactions, interventions provided, and the patients response to those interventions
- teaching provided to the patient and family, their understanding of the teaching, and if follow-up teaching is needed.

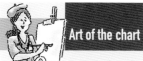

Art of the chart

Assisting with bone marrow aspiration

Here's an example of how to document assisting with a bone marrow aspiration procedure.

5/3/2017	1015	Dr. K. Wallace in to perform bone marrow aspiration. Informed consent
		obtained. Education provided regarding procedure and all questions an
		swered. Pt stated understanding of procedure. Pt positioned on R side.
		Time-out performed (see Time-out documentation sheet). Pt sedated
		with 4 mg midazolam I.V. (see eMAR) Aspiration performed on L iliac
		crest. Specimen obtained and sent to lab. Bone marrow site w/o signs of
		bleeding. Band-Aid in place. Vital signs stable throughout (see vital signs
		sheet). Pt tolerated procedure well. Pain rated as "0" on scale of 0 to 10.
		————————————————————— P. Clark RN

If your EHR has specific screens designated for procedures, be sure to utilize them correctly. If not using an EHR, complete a nurses' note describing the procedure and the patient's condition. (See Assisting with bone marrow aspiration.)

Esophageal tube insertion and removal

After assisting the practitioner with esophageal tube insertion or removal, document:
- date and time that you assisted in the insertion or removal
- name of the practitioner who performed the procedure
- type of esophageal tube inserted
- intragastric balloon pressure; amount of air injected into the gastric balloon port; amount of fluid used for gastric irrigation; and color, consistency, and amount of gastric return before and after lavage (if applicable)
- baseline intraesophageal balloon pressure, which varies with respirations and esophageal contractions
- patient's tolerance of the insertion and removal procedures
- patient's vital signs before, during, and after the procedure.

If your EHR has specific screens designated for esophageal tubes, which may be part of the GI assessment screens, be sure to utilize them correctly. If not using an EHR, complete a nurses' note describing the procedure and the patient's condition.

Arterial line insertion and removal

When assisting a practitioner who's inserting an arterial line, document:
- date and time of insertion
- practitioner's name
- insertion site
- type, gauge, and length of the catheter
- patient teaching, understanding of the teaching, and if follow-up teaching is needed
- patient's response to the procedure, including circulation status to the involved extremity.

The arterial line's work may be done, but not yours . . .

Document ongoing use and care, which includes:
- calibration and zeroing of equipment per unit policy and procedure
- blood pressure readings
- that alarm limits are set appropriately for the patient's current condition and that the alarms are turned on, functioning properly, and audible to staff
- site assessment, including signs of infection, bleeding, or fluid leakage
- site care, dressing change, and tubing change.
  After removing the arterial line, document:
- date and time the catheter was discontinued
- length of the catheter
- condition of the insertion site
- specimens that were obtained from the catheter for culture, if applicable
- patient's response to the procedure
- amount of time pressure was held at site.
  If your EHR has specific screens designated for arterial lines, which may be part of the I.V. documentation screens, be sure to utilize them correctly. If not using an EHR, complete a nurses' note describing the procedure and monitoring as well as the patient's condition.

CVAD insertion and removal

When you assist the practitioner to insert a CVAD, you need to document:
- time and date of insertion
- practitioner's name
- the time-out conducted before the procedure started, including who was involved in the time-out, and the confirmation of the

Art of the chart

Assisting with central venous access device insertion

Here's an example of how to document assisting with a central venous access device (CVAD).

6/6/2017	1030	Procedure explained to pt who stated understanding. Informed consent
		obtained by Dr. E. Rafferty. TLC placed on 1st attempt via R subclavian vein.
		All ports flushed with 10 ml NSS after blood return confirmed. Sutured
		in place. Chest X-ray ordered. Pt tolerated procedure well. VS stable
		throughout (see VS sheet). ————————————————— E. Ryan, RN

right patient, right site, procedure and, as applicable, all relevant information and necessary equipment were available
- type, length, and location of the access device
- patient's response to the procedure
- time that X-rays were performed to confirm correct placement, the results, and when you notified the practitioner of confirmation. Also document if more than one attempt was made to insert.
- solutions or medications infusing
- patient and family (if applicable) teaching, their understanding of your teaching, and if follow-up teaching is needed.
  If your EHR has specific screens designated for central lines, which may be part of the I.V. documentation screens, be sure to utilize them correctly. If not using an EHR, complete a nurses' note describing the procedure and monitoring as well as the patient's condition. (See Assisting with central venous access device insertion.)
  Document ongoing use and care, which includes:
- site assessment, including signs of infection, bleeding, or fluid leakage
- site care, dressing change, and tubing change
- blood return from CVAD ports assessed per facility policy and procedure
- flushing of ports, if applicable.

Out with the access device, in with the documenting . . .

After removal of a CVAD, document:
- time and date of removal and the patient's response
- type of dressing applied
- condition of the insertion site
- catheter specimens you collected for culture or other analysis.

Lumbar puncture

When you assist the practitioner who performs a lumbar puncture, document:
- time and date of procedure
- practitioner's name
- the time-out conducted before the procedure started, including who was involved in the time-out, and the confirmation of the right patient, right site, procedure and, as applicable, all relevant information and necessary equipment were available
- color and clarity of the fluid obtained
- number of test tubes sent to the laboratory for analysis
- how the patient tolerated the procedure
- patient and family (if applicable) teaching, their understanding of your teaching, and if follow-up teaching is needed
- your interventions and care after the procedure, including keeping the patient in a supine position for 6 to 12 hours; encouraging fluid intake; and assessing for headache, pain, and leaking cerebrospinal fluid around the puncture site
- signs of complications, such as a change in LOC, dizziness, or changes in vital signs; the date, time, and practitioner who was notified; interventions provided; and the patient's response to those interventions.

If your EHR has specific screens designated for procedures, be sure to utilize them correctly. If not using an EHR, complete a nurses' note describing the procedure, specimens sent to the lab, as well as the patient's condition.

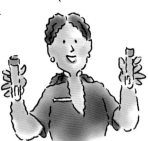

When documenting lumbar puncture, record how many test tubes were sent for analysis.

Paracentesis

When you assist the practitioner who performs a paracentesis, document:
- date and time of the procedure
- practitioner's name
- the time-out conducted before the procedure started, including who was involved in the time-out, and the confirmation of the right patient, right site, procedure and, as applicable, all relevant information and necessary equipment were available
- puncture site
- whether the site was sutured
- amount, color, viscosity, and odor of the initially aspirated fluid (also, record this in the I&O record)
- patient and family (if applicable) teaching, their understanding of your teaching, and if follow-up teaching is needed.

With responsibility comes more documentation

If you're responsible for ongoing patient care, document:
- running record of the patient's vital signs per facility protocol
- frequency of drainage checks per facility protocol
- patient's response to the paracentesis
- characteristics of the drainage, including color, amount, odor, and viscosity
- patient's daily weight and abdominal girth measurements (taken at about the same time every day)
- what fluid specimens were sent to the laboratory for analysis
- signs of complications, such as peritoneal fluid leakage or abdominal pain. Also document the date, time, and practitioner who was notified; interventions provided; and the patient's response to those interventions.

If your EHR has specific screens designated for a paracentesis, which may be part of the GI documentation screens, be sure to utilize them correctly. If not using an EHR, complete a nurses' note describing the procedure and monitoring as well as the patient's condition.

Thoracentesis

When assisting the practitioner who is performing a thoracentesis, you need to document:
- date and time of the procedure
- name of the practitioner who performed it
- the time-out conducted before the procedure started, including who was involved in the time-out, and the confirmation of the right patient, right site, procedure and, as applicable, all relevant information and necessary equipment were available
- amount and characteristics of fluid aspirated
- fluid specimens sent to the laboratory for analysis
- patient's response to the procedure
- patient and family (if applicable) teaching, their understanding of your teaching, and if follow-up teaching is needed
- complications, such as sudden or unusual pain, faintness, dizziness, changes in vital signs, symptoms of pneumothorax, hemothorax, subcutaneous emphysema, or infection. Document the date, time, and name of the practitioner notified; the interventions provided; and the patient's response to those interventions.

If your EHR has specific screens designated for thoracentesis, which may be part of the respiratory documentation screens, be sure to utilize them correctly. If not using an EHR, complete a nurses' note describing the procedure and monitoring as well as the patient's condition.

Documenting miscellaneous procedures

Documentation isn't limited to procedures you perform or help the practitioner perform. You'll also document other situations, including the ones described here.

Diagnostic tests

Before receiving a diagnosis, the patient may undergo diagnostic testing, such as a magnetic resonance imaging (MRI) or cardiac catheterization. Your patient assessment and care associated with these tests should be included in the patient's medical record.

Document your first impressions

Start your documentation by recording preliminary assessments you made of the patient's condition. For example, if the patient is pregnant or has allergies, these conditions might affect the way a test is performed or the test's result. If the patient's age, illness, or disability requires special preparation for a test, record this information as well.

Document what education was provided to the patient and family (if applicable) about the test and follow-up care, the administration or withholding of drugs and preparations, special diets, food or fluid restrictions, enemas, and specimen collection. Be sure to document their understanding of what was taught and if additional teaching is needed.

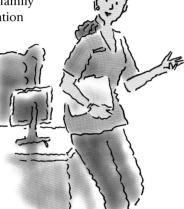

When documenting a diagnostic test, begin by recording your preliminary assessment findings.

Paperwork??

Some tests require additional documentation of the patient's condition, such as the verification that the patient does not have metal in the body prior to a MRI. Become familiar with the paperwork required by your facility before sending a patient for a diagnostic test in order to avoid unnecessary complications or delay in care.

Pain control

Pain control is a priority concern for most patients. According to The Joint Commission standards, facilities need to utilize methods to assess a patient's pain according to the patient's age, condition, and ability to understand. In your quest to eliminate, minimize, or control your patient's pain, you may use a number of assessment tools to determine the degree of pain. When you use these tools, always document the results. (See *Document pain three ways*, page 183.)

When documenting pain levels and characteristics, determine whether the pain is internal, external, localized, or diffuse and

Document pain three ways

Some facilities use standardized questionnaires, such as the McGill Pain Questionnaire or the Initial Pain Assessment Tool. Other facilities have devised their own pain measurement tools, such as the flow sheet and rating scales shown below. Whichever pain assessment tool your facility utilizes, remember to document the results of the assessment and the tool utilized, if needed.

Pain flow sheet

Flow sheets are convenient tools for pain assessment because they allow documentation of your reassessment of the patient's pain at appropriate intervals. They're also useful when patients and families feel too overwhelmed to answer a long, detailed questionnaire.

PAIN FLOW SHEET

Record the patient's pain rating before medication administration here.

	Pain rating (0 to 10)	Patient behaviors	Vital signs	Pain rating after intervention	Interventions
D17 0800	7	Wincing, holding head	BP 186/88 HR 98- RR 22		Dilaudid 2 mg I.M. given
11/20/2017 1200	3	Relaxing, reading	BP 160/80 HR 84- RR 18	2	

Record the patient's pain rating after interventions provided here.

Visual analog pain scale

With a visual analog pain scale, the patient marks a linear scale at the point that corresponds to the perceived degree of pain. The typical scale shown below uses the phrases "no pain" at one end and "pain as bad as it could be" at the other end.

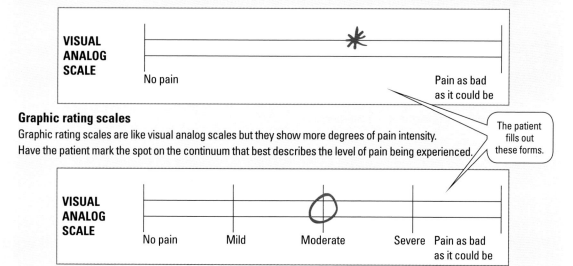

VISUAL ANALOG SCALE — No pain / Pain as bad as it could be

Graphic rating scales

Graphic rating scales are like visual analog scales but they show more degrees of pain intensity. Have the patient mark the spot on the continuum that best describes the level of pain being experienced.

The patient fills out these forms.

VISUAL ANALOG SCALE — No pain / Mild / Moderate / Severe / Pain as bad as it could be

whether it interferes with the patient's sleep or other activities of daily living. Document how the patient describes the pain in the medical record using the patient's own words in "parentheses." Also assess and document the patient's expectations of pain control. For example, a patient undergoing a total knee replacement may expect pain to be controlled at a level "3" on a scale of 0 to 10.

Translating body language

Be aware of the patient's body language and behaviors associated with pain. Does the patient wince or grimace? Does the patient move or squirm in bed? Document measures that relieve or worsen the pain. Also, note if the pain appears to worsen or improve when visitors are present. Document interventions provided, including pain medications and how the patient responded.

If your EHR has specific screens designated for pain assessment and reassessment, be sure to utilize them correctly. If not using an EHR, complete a nurses' note describing the patient's pain, interventions provided, and effectiveness of those interventions. (See Pain assessment and reassessment documentation.)

Hourly rounding

Hourly rounding is a practice that has been shown to reduce call light use and increase patient safety and satisfaction by proactively meeting patient needs. Hourly rounding is commonly alternated between the primary nurse, ancillary staff, such as a certified nurse assistant, and at times, the charge nurse. Documentation of the hourly rounds, as well as interventions provided during rounding, may be completed using a

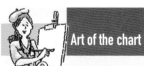

Art of the chart

Pain assessment and reassessment documentation

Here's an example of documentation of a patient's pain.

7/2/2017	0830	Pt complaining of lower back pain. Pt rates pain as "8" on scale 0 to 10.
		Describes pain as a continuous ache that worsens with movement.
		Pt repositioned for comfort. Observed pt wincing with movement. ————
		————————————————————————————————— S. Bane, RN
7/2/2017	0845	Pt given morphine sulfate 2 mg I.V. ———————————— S. Bane, RN
7/2/2017	0915	Pt reassessed for pain. States pain level of "3" on scale 0 to 10. Resting
		in bed watching TV. ———————————————————— S. Bane, RN

flow sheet, rounding log (facility-created form), or through use of the EHR. Documentation should include:

- date and time of rounding
- interventions provided, such as repositioning the patient or providing pain medication
- patient response to interventions
- teaching provided to patient or family.

I&O

Many patients, including critical care patients; surgical and burn patients; those receiving I.V. therapy; and those with fluid and electrolyte imbalances, hemorrhage, or edema need 24-hour I&O monitoring. To expedite documentation, you'll probably keep I&O sheets at the bedside or by the bathroom door; however, be sure to transfer this information to either the EHR or the I&O flow sheet in the patient's medical record. If the patient is incontinent, document this as well as tube drainage and irrigation volumes. Teach family members the importance of notifying you if they empty urinals or bedpans or if they assist the patient with eating.

Taking the intake documentation challenge

Keeping track of foods and fluids that are premeasured is easy. You can list the volumes of specific containers for quick reference and use infusion devices to more accurately record enteral and I.V. intake.

Keeping track of intake that isn't premeasured is more difficult. For example, measuring and recording a food such as gelatin that's fluid at room temperature requires the cooperation of the patient and other caregivers.

Don't forget these types of intake

Don't forget to document as intake I.V. piggyback infusions, drugs given by I.V. push, patient-controlled analgesics, and irrigation solutions that aren't withdrawn. Also, document oral or I.V. fluids that the patient receives when the patient is not on your unit. Doing so requires the cooperation of the patient and staff members in other departments. In addition, remind the ambulatory patient to use a urinal, commode, or collection container placed in the bathroom.

Fluid loss through the GI tract is normally 100 ml or less daily. However, if the patient's stools become excessive or watery, you should document them as output. Vomiting, drainage

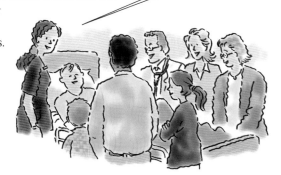

Keeping track of intake is a group effort! It requires the cooperation of the patient, family and friends, and your colleagues.

from suction devices and wound drains, and bleeding are other measurable sources of fluid loss that require documentation.

Transferring a patient to a specialty unit

If your patient's condition deteriorates and requires transfer to a specialty unit, be sure to document:

- date and time of a rapid response team call, if applicable (See *Rapid response team documentation.*)
- interventions provided related to the patient's condition and the patient's response to those interventions
- the transfer order for the level of care needed
- patient's condition at the time of transfer, including vital signs, descriptions of incisions and wounds, and locations of tubes or medical devices still in place as well as significant events during the hospital stay, noting whether the patient has advanced directives and special factors, such as allergies, a special diet, sensory deficits, and language or cultural issues

Rapid response team documentation

A rapid response team (RRT), also known as a *medical emergency* team, is a group of specially trained health care providers who respond to calls for deterioration in patient conditions with the goal of preventing cardiopulmonary arrest. Documentation is an important aspect of this care as it communicates to multidisciplinary team members the events that occurred, interventions provided, and the patient's response to those interventions. Documentation of a RRT call should include:

- date and time of the call
- name of the person who initiated the call
- names of the responders
- time the responders arrived
- reason for the call
- assessment findings
- verification of review of patient history and medications administered
- name of the practitioner notified
- testing performed and results
- interventions or medications administered
- patient response to interventions
- transfer to higher level of care (if ordered) or indicated
- notification of the unit the patient is being transferred to
- hand-off communication provided to receiving nurse
- notification of the family regarding event and transfer (if applicable).

- medications, treatments, and teaching needs, noting which goals were and weren't met
- time that you gave a report to the receiving unit, including the name of the nurse who received the report
- date and time of the transfer, along with how the patient was transported to the specialty unit and who accompanied the patient
- any patient teaching related to the transfer such as the reason for transfer
- notification of family regarding the transfer.

Withdrawal of life support

According to the right-to-die laws of most states, a patient has the right to refuse extraordinary life-supporting measures if there is no hope of recovery. If the patient can't make the decision, the patient's next of kin is usually permitted to decide if life support should continue. A written statement of the patient's wishes is always preferable.

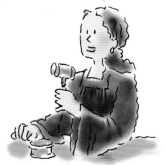

The Patient Self-Determination Act requires that the patient be asked upon admission about having an advance directive.

Advanced warning

Because of the Patient Self-Determination Act, each health care facility is required to ask the patient upon admission if an advance directive exists. An advance directive is a statement of the patient's wishes if the patient is unable to make decisions regarding care. An advance directive may include a living will, which goes into effect when the patient can't make decisions regarding care, as well as a durable health care power of attorney, which names a designated person to make these decisions when the patient can't. The act also states that the patient must receive written information concerning the right to make decisions about medical care. (See chapter 6, Avoiding legal pitfalls.)

Match the patient's wishes to the situation

If life support is to be withdrawn, read the patient's advance directive to ensure that the present situation matches the patient's wishes and verify that the risk manager has reviewed the document if complex issues are present. If the patient does not have an advance directive, ensure that the patient (if able) and family have discussed all options for care with the practitioner before making the final decision to withdrawal care. Provide teaching to the family and patient (if able) regarding what to expect when life-support is discontinued and answer all questions. Check that the appropriate consent forms have been signed. Ask the family whether they would like spiritual support present and if they would like to be with the patient before, during, and after withdrawal of care.

Before withdrawal of life support

When it has been decided to withdraw life support, be sure to document:

- if the patient's advance directive matches the present situation and life support wishes
- that your facility's risk manager has reviewed the advance directive if complex issues are present
- the practitioner who spoke with the patient and family and entered the order for withdrawal of life support
- that a consent form has been signed to withdraw life support, according to facility policy
- the names of persons who were notified of the decision to withdraw life support and their responses
- any teaching provided to the patient and family regarding the process and their understanding of the teaching
- medication administered, such as sedation or pain medication and patient response.

After withdrawal of life support, be sure to document:

- time of withdrawal of life support
- types of physical care provided to the patient before and after life support withdrawal
- whether the family was with the patient before, during, and after withdrawal of life support as well as person who is present for spiritual support; document notification of the family if they were not present
- the time the patient expired and who made the pronouncement

Note: Practitioners may designate an RN to pronounce a patient if the RN has completed the necessary education and competency to do so.

- family's response, your interventions for them, and after-care for the patient
- date and time of notification of the patient's expiration to the area organ donor center per state law and facility policy and procedure
- date and time of notification of the patient's expiration to the practitioners involved in patient's care
- name of mortuary and the time of notification and patient pick-up if the patient expires.

Note: Document if, after withdrawal of life support, the patient was transferred to another unit, such as a hospice unit.

If your EHR has specific screens designated for withdrawal of life support, be sure to utilize them correctly. If not using an EHR, complete a nurses' note describing the event, including education provided to patient and family, their understanding of the situation, interventions provided, and outcomes of those interventions. If the patient expires, be sure to document on the appropriate screens or document for notifications and disposition of the patient's body. (See Withdrawal of life support documentation, page 189.)

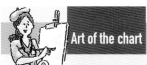

Art of the chart

Withdrawal of life support documentation

2/2/2017	1800	Pt's wife, Joan, discussed withdrawal of care with Dr. P. Reed. Pt's advance
		directive in chart. Pt presently unresponsive to pain. Consent for with
		drawal of care signed. Education provided to Joan regarding what to
		expect when life support is removed. All questions answered. Joan's sister
		also present. Morphine drip started at 5 mg/hr per Dr. Reed. —— L. Danios, RN
2/2/2017	1900	Endotracheal tube removed by J. Chavez, RT. O₂ at 4L via nasal cannula.
		Wife at bedside. ———————————————— L. Danios, RN
2/2/2017	2030	Pt without respirations. Cardiac monitor shows asystole. Unable to obtain
		pulse. Pt pronounced by charge nurse, M. Davy, RN. Morphine drip
		discontinued. Wife remains at bedside. ———————— L. Danois, RN
2/2/2017	2100	Postmortem care provided. Dr. P. Reed notified of pt expiration. Organ
		donor center notified. Wife to provide mortuary information by 2130.
		———————————————————— L. Danois, RN

Codes

Guidelines established by the American Heart Association direct you to keep a documented, chronologic account of a patient's condition and events throughout a code situation. This documentation may occur on a paper form or through use of a computer. If you're the designated recorder during a code, document therapeutic interventions and the patient's responses *as* they occur. Don't rely on your memory later.

> During a code situation, a designated recorder should document events as they occur.

Getting up to code

The form or computer screen used to document a code situation is the *code record*. It incorporates detailed information about who participated in the code, time of all interventions performed, patient's condition (including cardiac rhythm) and response to those interventions as well as time and dosage of medications administered. Outcome of the code is also documented, such as transfer of the patient to a higher level of care, if applicable, or termination of the code. The code record is signed by the recorder and the practitioner who directed the code. Cardiac rhythm strips printed during the code situation are placed in the patient's medical record. (See *Documenting a code situation*, page 190.)

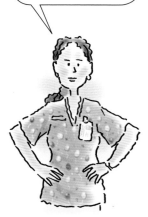

Documenting a code situation

A completed code record like the one below should be included in your patient's chart.

CODE RECORD

Pg. _/_ of _/_

Arrest Date: _1/9/17_
Arrest Time: _0631_
Rm/Location: _431-2_
Discovered by:
C. Brown
☑ RN ☐ MD
☐ Other

Methods of alert:
☐ Witnessed, monitored: rhythm
☐ Witnessed, unmonitored
☑ Unwitnessed, unmonitored
☐ Unwitnessed, monitored; rhythm
Diagnosis: _Post anterior wall MI_

Condition when found:
☑ Unresponsive
☐ Apneic
☐ Pulseless
☐ Hemorrhage
☐ Seizure

Ventilation management:
Time: _0635_
Method:
oral ET tube
Precordial thump:
CPR initiated at:
_0631_

Previous airway:
☐ ET tube
☐ Trach
☑ Natural

Addressograph

CPR PROGRESS NOTES

Time	Pulse CPR	Resp. rate Spont; bag	Blood pressure	Rhythm	Defib (joules)	Atropine	Epinephrine	Amiodarone	ACTIONS/PATIENT RESPONSE — Responses to therapy, procedures, labs drawn/results
							I.V. PUSH	INFUSIONS	
0632	No pulse CPR	Bag	0	V fib	200				No change.
0633	No pulse CPR	Bag	0	V fib	200		1 mg		No change
0635	40	Bag	60 palp	SB PVCs					Oral intubation by Dr. David Hart
0645	60	Bag	80/40	SB PVCs					ABGs drawn. Ⓡ fem pressure applied.

ABGs & Lab Data

Time Spec Sent	pH	PCO	Po₂	HCO₃−	Sat%	Fio₂	Other
0653	7.1	76	43	14	80%		

Resuscitation outcome
☑ Successful ☑ Transferred to _ccu_ at _0700_
☐ Unsuccessful — Expired at ____
Pronounced by: ____ MD
Family notified by: _S. Quinn, RN_
Time: _0645_
Attending notified by: _S. Quinn, RN_ Time _0645_
Code Recorder _S. Quinn, RN_
Code Team Nurse _B. Mullen, RN_
Anesthesia Rep. _J. Hanna, RN_
Other Personnel _Dr. Hart_
B. Russo, RT
Signature _Connie Brown, RN Recorder_

A helpful critique

Some facilities use a *resuscitation critique* form to identify actual or potential problems with the resuscitation process. This form tracks personnel responses and response times as well as the availability of appropriate drugs and functioning equipment. Make sure that a copy of the completed critique form is submitted to the appropriate department or code committee for analysis.

That's a wrap!

Documenting procedures review

Documentation regarding procedures includes most of the same elements, whether performing the procedure or assisting with the procedure. These elements include:

• what procedure was performed
• when it was performed
• who performed it
• how it was performed
• how well the patient tolerated it
• teaching provided to the patient and family, their understanding of that teaching, and if follow-up teaching is needed
• complications from the procedure, if any, name of the practitioner notified, interventions provided, and the patient's response to those intervention.

For procedures that require consent, such as a bone marrow aspiration or lumbar puncture, be sure to verify that a consent was signed and is in the patient's medical record. For most invasive procedures, be sure to document the time-out conducted before the procedure started, including who was involved in the time-out, and the confirmation of the right patient, right site, procedure, and, as applicable, all relevant information and necessary equipment were available. Also, be sure to document any specimens obtained.

Documenting miscellaneous procedures

• Document all diagnostic tests a patient receives and how they were tolerated.
• Use an assessment tool to determine the degree of pain your patient is experiencing.
• Document specific procedures, such as hourly rounding and intake and output on facility forms.
• Document transferring your patient to a specialty unit if the patient's condition deteriorates.
• Document withdrawal of life support, per patient and family wishes.
• Document a code situation using a specific code record to allow a chronologic account of a patient's condition, interventions, and outcome of a code.

Suggested references

American Association of Critical-Care Nurses. "AACN Practice Alert: Alarm Management," 2013. Available: http://ccn.aacnjournals.org/content/33/5/83.full.pdf (Level VII).

American Nurse's Association. Principles for Documentation. American Nurses Association, 2010.

Carpenito, L.J. *Nursing Care Plans: Transitional Patient & Family Centered Care (Nursing Care Plans & Documentation)*, 7th ed. Philadelphia, PA: Lippincott Williams & Wilkins, 2017.

Halm, M.A. "Hourly Rounds: What Does the Evidence Indicate?" *American Journal of Critical Care* 18(6): 581-584, November 2009.

Institute for Safe Medication Practices. "Independent Double-Checks: Undervalued and Misused". ISMP Medication Safety Alert! Nurse Advise-ERR, 12(3), 1, 2014. Available: http://www.ismp.org/newsletters/nursing/issues /NurseAdviseERR201403.pdf (Level VII).

Institute for Safe Medication Practices. "Side Tracks on the Safety Express: Interruptions Lead to Errors and Unfinished . . . Wait, What Was I doing?" Nurse Advise-ERR, 11(2), 1–4, 2012. Available: https://www.ismp.org/Newsletters /acutecare/showarticle.aspx?id=37 (Level VII).

The Joint Commission. "Joint Commission Statement on Pain Management," 2016. Available: https://www.jointcommission.org/joint_commission_statement _on_pain_management/.

The Joint Commission. *Standard NPSG.01.01.01: Comprehensive Accreditation Manual for Hospitals*. Oakbrook Terrace, IL: The Joint Commission, 2018.

The Joint Commission. *Standard RC.02.01.01: Comprehensive Accreditation Manual for Hospitals*. Oakbrook Terrace, IL: The Joint Commission, 2018. (Level VII).

Chapter 8

Documenting special situations

Just the facts

In this chapter, you'll learn:

◆ special situations related to patient rights and safety and the way nurses should respond to them

◆ special situations that affect personal safety and the way nurses should respond to them

◆ the proper way to document each of these special situations.

A look at special situations

Although proper documentation is essential in all areas of health care, it plays a key role in protecting patient rights and ensuring patient safety in special situations. Thorough and objective documentation can also be effective in situations that affect the nurse's safety and well-being in the workplace.

Situations related to patient rights and safety

Depending on your area of practice, you may need to:
- request permission to photograph a patient
- request permission for information to be released to the media
- search for contraband
- document instances of equipment tampering.
  You'll need to document each of these special situations accordingly while protecting patient rights and ensuring patient safety.

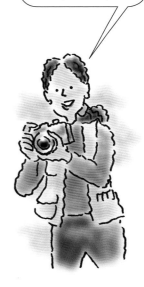

Don't take off that lens cap unless you have permission from the patient to take the photograph.

Photographing a patient

Photographs placed into the medical record are important to memorialize and provide evidence of certain patient conditions and can be used in court proceedings. For example, to document patient outcomes related to trends in wound healing or documentation of injuries that may have occurred prior to or during hospitalization. Photographs may also be commonly taken of child abuse, rape, or accident victims to document the severity of the injury and to serve as proof that the injury occurred. What is important to remember is to document and photograph, if applicable, all conditions the patient presents with prior to admission versus conditions that occurred during hospitalization, otherwise known as "hospital acquired" for which the hospital and you as the caregiver can be liable for. Also, be sure to document that you took a photograph in the medical record so that anyone reviewing the medical record is aware that one was taken.

Get the old John Hancock

Photographs of patients fall under the Health Insurance Portability and Accountability Act (HIPAA) of 1996. Unless state and federal laws specify otherwise (some states have special laws for forensic cases), the patient must provide informed consent to be photographed. (See *Permission to photograph*, page 195.) Some facilities have decided to embed consent to photograph into other documents such as the "conditions of admission" or "surgical procedure consents." Keep in mind, however, that a health care facility can decide to not photograph the patient if this will interfere with the delivery of care to the patient, even if the patient has provided consent. Become familiar with your facility's policy and/or state laws related to taking photographs so that you keep you and your facility out of any legal trouble.

What is my role with photographs?

Your facility's policy and procedure for photographing patients should outline the following:

- circumstances defining when and how patient photography is allowed at your facility
- patient-consent processes, including who is responsible for obtaining the consent
- who owns the photographic images (facilities almost always retain copyright ownership)
- how images are stored and retrieved. All photographs need to be securely stored in a way that will allow easy access to appropriate caregivers, preserve the photograph's quality, and protect the patient's privacy.
- record retention—how long images are kept—should follow the same time frames as any other part of the medical record
- when, why, and to whom patients may authorize release and use of images outside of the facility's jurisdiction.

Some other things to consider: Only use equipment that is authorized by your facility to take these types of patient pictures. For example, facilities usually have designated cameras that must be used to take photos. Never use your own personal camera or phone to take patient pictures as this violates patient privacy.

Permission to photograph

Depending on your facility's policy and procedure, you may use a form similar to this one to obtain permission to photograph a patient.

Permission to photograph and release of photograph

Date *3/25/2017*

I hereby give my permission for a photograph to be taken of *wound*

This photograph is being taken for the following purpose(s): *to monitor wound healing progression*

I intend to be legally bound hereby.

Angela Steiner   Signed *Barry Arnold*
(Witness)

                                    Address *771 Holly Drive*
                                             Philadelphia, PA

If the patient is unable to sign or is a minor, complete the following:

Patient is a minor who is _____ years of age and whose date of birth is
_____, or the patient is unable to sign because:
        (month, day, and year)

_____   _____
        (Witness)   (Closest Relative or Guardian)

No signature required

Signed consent isn't required for photographs of personal or family situations that don't involve the health care facility as these photos are not part of the medical record. Examples include taking pictures of a new baby or a birthday celebration.

Permanent fixture

Photographs that do require permission to be taken become a permanent part of the patient's medical record. Follow your facility's policy and procedure on obtaining patient consent, and document that pictures were taken in the medical record if you are the one who took the photographs or are involved with the process.

> Photos relating to the patient's care become part of the medical record.

Releasing information to the media

Patient confidentiality continues to be a priority of health care workers and patients. When seeking health care services, the patient trusts that the information shared with a health care provider will remain confidential. Those who come in contact with a patient in a health care setting have a legal and ethical obligation to maintain confidentiality and adhere to guidelines outlined in the HIPAA. HIPAA has established a minimum acceptable threshold for the use and release of patient's health information. Under HIPAA privacy regulations, patients must be informed about how their "protected health information" (PHI) will be used and given the opportunity to object to or restrict the use or release of their information. This would include release of information to the public, including the media. However, hospitals may use and disclose PHI without a patient's consent for purposes of treatment, payment, and health care operations. HIPAA also specifically requires that each hospital adopt and implement written policies and procedures that are designed to ensure its compliance with the HIPAA Privacy Rule.

Permission policy

Unless a patient objects, the following limited information can be placed in a hospital directory and released to the public, including the media, when someone specifically asks about a patient by name:
- patient's name
- patient's location in the facility
- patient's condition, described in standardized general terms that do not communicate specific information about the individual
- patient's religious affiliation (may only be released to clergy—clergy do not have to inquire about a patient by name).

Any other information, including detailed statements regarding a specific patient's care and treatment, photographs, or interviews, require written permission from the patient or legal representative. Therefore, each health care facility should have policies and procedures in place for handling all types of media requests for specific patient information. If permission to release information by the patient or legal representative is granted, only people designated and trained to disclose information to the media should be allowed to do so. All of these details should be outlined in the facility's policies and procedures.

One-word is enough

The American Hospital Association has suggested the following "one-word" descriptions of a patient's general condition:
- undetermined—patient awaiting physician assessment
- good—patient is stable; indicators are excellent

- fair—patient is stable; indicators are favorable
- serious—patient is acutely ill; indicators are questionable
- critical—patient may be unconscious; indicators are unfavorable.

In the spotlight

If the situation involves a well-known patient (someone who is in the public eye, such as a celebrity, or is newsworthy because of the nature of the condition), releasing information to the media on a regular basis may be in the patient's best interest. Without a formal statement, the media can easily distort situation and condition of the patient.

The practitioner and the patient or legal representative should agree on what information should be included in the statement, thus ensuring an accurate, mutually agreed upon, release of information. This information may then be released to the media by the designated facility spokesperson.

Documenting duties

Before a patient's information may be released to the media, make sure the patient (or legal representative) has provided written consent.

Documentation in the nurses' notes should reflect consent from the patient and practitioner to release information to the media. If the nurse assists the facility spokesperson in obtaining information or consent, this should also be documented in the nurses' notes. Remember to include the date, time, and name of the facility spokesperson in the note. Be sure to follow your facility's policies and procedures for media releases. (See *Permission to release information to the media.*)

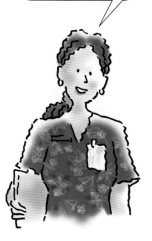

Releasing formal statements to the media about a patient's condition ensures that the information is accurate and mutually agreed upon by the practitioner and the patient or legal representative.

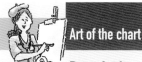

Art of the chart

Permission to release information to the media

This example illustrates how to document whether a patient has given permission to release information to the media.

4/1/2017	1300	Pt. granted permission to Dr. W. Jones, attending physician, and Anita Robinson,
		public relations, to release a statement to the media regarding her condition.
		States, "All inquiries and/or calls are to be handled by Anita Robinson and her
		staff." Assured pt. her wishes would be honored and respected. ————————
		———————————————————————————————————— J. Brown, RN
4/1/2017	1315	Dr. W. Jones placed order in chart reflecting his permission for
		Anita Robinson, public relations, to release his name to the media. ————
		———————————————————————————————————— J. Brown, RN

For the (public) record

Patients involved in matters of public record have the very same privacy rights as all other patients. This means that as long as the patient has not requested that information be withheld, you can release the patient's one-word condition and location to individuals who inquire about the patient by name. This also includes certain types of cases, such as police, coroner cases, or child abuse cases which require reporting to government agencies. The fact that a hospital is required to report certain confidential information to a government agency does not make that information public, meaning you still need patient consent to release information. However, in disaster situations, hospitals may disclose information regarding a patient's health to a public or private entity authorized by law to assist in disaster relief efforts.

Dealing with death

When a patient death occurs, the facility may release that information to the media after the patient's family and next of kin have been notified. Additionally, the hospital should also report the death as required by law. Information about the date, time, and cause of death must come from the patient's practitioner, and the patient's legal representative must approve its release. If the death is suspicious in nature, all inquiries must be forwarded to the appropriate coroner. (See *Nonreleasable patient information*.)

Searching for contraband

Contraband is defined as any item that's prohibited from being in the patient's possession while in the facility. Examples may include:
- controlled substances
- drug paraphernalia
- alcohol
- weapons (such as firearms, knives, explosive agents, or chemical agents).

Probable cause?

Searching a patient's possessions for contraband is appropriate only when there's clear evidence that a patient may possess a substance or object that may harm the patient or others. If you suspect that a patient has a dangerous substance or object, notify your nurse-manager and the security department immediately. You may be directed to ask the patient to disclose the possession of the contraband. If the patient doesn't disclose possession of the items, you need the patient's permission to search personal belongings.

Nonreleasable patient information

Under certain circumstances, a hospital has an obligation to report certain confidential information to government agencies. However, this does not make that information public and available to the media. Patient information regarding the following topics typically cannot be released to the media even with consent from the patient (state laws may vary so become familiar with the laws in your state):
- substance abuse
- psychiatric admission
- sexual assault
- suicide or attempted suicide
- child, spouse, or elderly abuse
- rare diseases or reportable genetic anomalies
- HIV status
- sexually transmitted diseases.

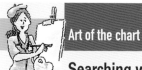

Art of the chart

Searching without permission

Here's an example of how to document a search conducted without the patient's permission.

5/7/2017	1100	Pt stated, "I have a switchblade—so no one had better mess with me."
		Pt refuses for staff to search belongings. ——————— K. Owens, RN
5/7/2017	1105	Security called. Nurse-manager, E. Davy, RN and risk management director,
		A. Smith notified. ——————— K. Owens, RN
5/7/2017	1110	Tom Jones, security, reported to room. Pt's backpack confiscated and
		black-handled switchblade retrieved. Education provided to patient regarding
		safety of patients and staff. Switchblade placed hospital safe until
		discharge. Pt states "Ok, I understand." ——————— K. Owens, RN

Request denied

If a patient denies the request for a search and you still suspect that the patient has dangerous contraband, notify the proper authorities so they can evaluate whether a search is necessary. This usually includes the attending practitioner, the risk management department, and an administrator of the health care facility. (See *Searching without permission*.)

Can I have a witness?

If a search is required, request to have someone present to witness the search and follow your facility's policy for searching for contraband.

Search basics

Here are some guidelines to consider when searching for contraband:
- Searches should take place in a private setting if possible.
- A nurse should be present during the search.
- The persons conducting the search should be of the same gender as the patient.
- Safety of the person performing the search should be considered. For example, wear appropriate personal protective equipment such as gloves and use a pen or pencil to sort through clothing to make sure no sharp objects are present.
- Unless an item poses a threat to the safety or well-being of the patient or staff, outside law enforcement agencies don't need to be contacted.

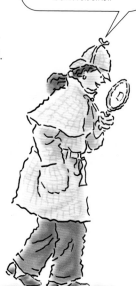

Don't request to search a patient's possessions unless you have clear evidence of contraband.

Take note

When documenting a search, include these items in the patient's record:
- identity of staff members present during the search
- reason for search
- reason for suspicion of contraband
- contraband's potential for causing harm to the patient or others
- items recovered during the search.

Equipment tampering

At times, a patient and/or family member may tamper with equipment or misuse supplies without understanding the consequences. For example, the patient or family member may press keys on a pump or monitor, detach tubing, or play with equipment switches. If your patient or family member misuses equipment, explain that this behavior can cause harm. Educate the patient or family member to call for help if there are any concerns about equipment not working properly.

> Documentation for equipment tampering should include what the patient did and how you handled the situation, including patient and family education.

Write on

When tampering or misuse occurs, document in the progress notes what you saw the patient or family member do (or what the patient or family told you) and how you responded to the situation. Most medical equipment, including intravenous (I.V.) pumps and feeding pumps, have lock-out capabilities, which prevent the patient from manipulating the machine and should be utilized when indicated. (See *Patient tampering.*)

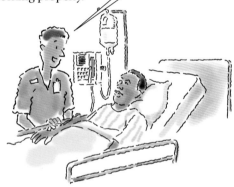

Art of the chart

Patient tampering

The notes below document a situation in which a patient tampered with equipment.

7/7/2017	0930	Found I.V. infusion of heparin off. Pt stated, "That alarm was annoying me,
		so I shut the machine off." Educated pt regarding importance of heparin
		drip and calling the nurse if an alarm goes off. Pt stated understanding.
		Call placed to Dr. J. Shaughnessy. ———————————— K. Conner, RN
7/7/2017	0945	Per Dr. J. Shaughnessy, stat PTT obtained. NSS infusing through I.V.
		catheter at 20 ml/hr. ———————————————— K. Conner, RN

Situations related to personal safety

In some cases, you'll need to document situations that affect your own safety and well-being in the workplace. Such situations include:
- hostile advances
- harassment, bullying, and sexual harassment.

Hostile advances

When a patient makes a hostile advance, the nurse's responsibility is to prevent harm to the patient, self, and others. The nurse should assess the emotional crisis or escalating behavior, provide emergency treatment to avoid worsening of the patient's condition, and objectively document the situation.

Take action

A sudden change in the patient's personality and/or escalating behavior can be a warning sign that the patient is becoming hostile. If a patient makes hostile advances, take these steps to intervene:
- Contain the patient in a safe environment. This may require assistance from staff members trained in crisis management to "deescalate" the patient's behavior.
- Follow facility guidelines for the use of restraints if necessary.
- Modify the environment. For example, place the patient in a private room, if possible, or decrease external stimulation.
- Designate a family member or staff member to provide one-to-one care of the patient. This means that the patient should be within eyesight and arm's length at all times. However, remain aware of the patient's right to privacy and dignity, especially during procedures and when the patient has to use the bathroom or a urinal, commode, or bedpan. The patient shouldn't be left alone during these times but should be protected from being exposed unnecessarily.
- Make frequent attempts to converse with the patient in a calm manner.
- Identify specific problem behaviors. Set limits and redirect any problem behavior.
- Set goals and reinforce appropriate behavior and conversation.
- Consider requesting a psychiatric consult.

The write stuff

Documentation should include a description of the patient's behavior and conversation and whether one-to-one observation is needed.

Record only the facts, not opinions, and quote patient statements, as indicated. Avoid labeling the patient. Be specific and objective in documentation. The need for ongoing one-to-one care should be documented according to your facility's policy but at a minimum each shift.

Harassment, bullying, and sexual harassment

In 2008, The Joint Commission issued a sentinel event alert which outlined a new leadership standard to address disruptive and inappropriate behavior, which mandated hospitals to have a code of conduct that defines acceptable, disruptive, and inappropriate behavior as well as the implementation of processes for managing these types of behaviors. The alert was updated in 2016 as these types of behaviors continue to undermine the culture of safety.

Harassment is defined as verbal or physical conduct that denigrates or shows aversion toward another individual based on race, culture, color, religion, gender, sexual orientation, national origin, age, or disability. Examples of harassing behaviors may include:
- derogatory comments or jokes
- slurs
- negative stereotyping
- interference with an individual's normal work
- derogatory posters, cartoon drawings, or electronically submitted e-mails.

Bullying may be described as repetitive, offensive, abusive, intimidating, or insulting behavior directed toward a person, including coworkers. Examples of bullying behaviors may include:
- harsh communication
- passive-aggressive behavior such as eye rolling, backstabbing, and scapegoating
- "silent" treatment
- withholding information
- failure to respect privacy.

The Equal Employment Opportunity Commission (EEOC) defines *sexual harassment* as "unwelcome sexual advances, requests for sexual favors, and other verbal or physical conduct of a sexual nature, when submission to or rejection of this conduct explicitly or implicitly affects an individual's employment; unreasonably interferes with an individual's work performance; or creates an intimidating, hostile, or offensive work environment." Examples of sexual harassment may include:
- repeated sexually oriented teasing or jokes
- flirtations

- sexual advances or propositions
- commentary about an individual's body
- whistling inappropriately
- touching, pinching, or brushing up against another's body
- displaying objects or pictures that are sexual in nature.

To be harassment free

Sexual harassment and harassment from a patient can be disturbing to a nurse. Even if the offending patient is elderly or cognitively impaired, distrust can develop between the patient and the nurse. The key is to maintain a professional relationship with the patient. Providing quality patient care should remain the utmost concern.

Whether it originates from a patient, a practitioner, another employee, an outside vendor, or a visitor, harassment and bullying in any form creates an intimidating and hostile work environment. Health care leaders have an obligation to provide an environment free from harassment and bullying, which is why reporting and documenting these types of behaviors is so important.

> Make sure that you document the facts, not your opinions.

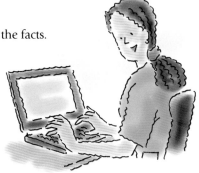

Focus on the facts

Documentation of this type of incident should include only the facts. Facilities may have a "zero tolerance" policy regarding inappropriate behavior and direct employees to complete a specific incident report to document the behavior of the harasser or bully. Don't include your perceptions, concerns, or thoughts regarding the specific behavior in the report. (See *Inappropriate behavior*.) All incidents of sexual harassment involving patients should also be reported per your facility's policies and procedures, which may include notifying the human resource or legal department.

Art of the chart

Inappropriate behavior

This example illustrates how to document inappropriate behavior.

1/15/2017	2100	Pt. pulled staff member onto bed and started kissing her. Discussed inappropriate behavior. Pt. unable to verbalize his understanding of conversation. ———————————————————— L. Green, RN

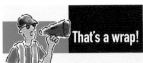

That's a wrap!

Documenting special situations review

Request to photograph a patient
• Become familiar with your facility's policy and/or state laws related to taking photographs.
• Photographs may commonly be taken in cases involving accidents, child abuse, or rape to memorialize and provide evidence of certain patient conditions.
• Signed consent usually is required prior to photographing the patient.
• Signed consent isn't required for photographs of personal or family situations that don't involve the health care facility as these photos are not part of the medical record.
• A health care facility can decide to not photograph the patient if this will interfere with delivering care to the patient, even if the patient has provided consent.

What to document
• Consent
• Photograph that was obtained

Release of information to the media
• Anyone who comes in contact with a patient in a health care facility is obliged to maintain confidentiality.
• Patients involved in matters of public record have the very same privacy rights as all other patients.
• Detailed statements regarding a specific patient's care and treatment, photographs, or interviews require written permission from the patient or legal representative.
• Patient information regarding certain topics, such as, substance abuse, HIV status, psychiatric admission, sexual assault, suicide, cases of child/spouse/elder abuse, rare diseases/reportable genetic anomalies, and sexually transmitted diseases typically cannot be released to the media even with consent from the patient.

What to document
• Consent from the patient or legal representative and practitioner
• Whether the nurse assisted the facility spokesperson in obtaining information or consent
• Date, time, and name of the facility spokesperson

Searching for contraband
• Contraband is any item that's prohibited from being in a patient's possession, such as controlled substances, drug paraphernalia, alcohol, and weapons.
• If a search is required, request to have someone present to witness the search and follow your facility's policy for searching for contraband.
• The search must be performed by someone of the same gender as the patient.

What to document
• Staff members present at search
• Reason for search
• Reason for suspicion of contraband
• Contraband's potential for causing harm to the patient or others
• Items recovered during the search

Equipment tampering
• The patient and/or family misuses or tampers with equipment.

What to document
• What you saw the patient or family do
• What you did about the situation
• Education provided to the patient or family regarding the incident

Hostile advances
• Safety of the patient and others is a priority.
• The patient must be contained in a safe environment.

What to document
• The behavior of the patient
• Whether one-to-one observation is needed
• The facts—not opinions, labels, or negative attitudes

Harassment and sexual harassment
• Health care leaders have obligation to provide an environment free from harassment.
• Harassment is verbal or physical conduct that denigrates or shows hostility or aversion toward another

Documenting special situations review *(continued)*

individual based on race, culture, color, religion, gender, sexual orientation, national origin, age, or disability.
• Sexual harassment is offensive, unwelcome, or unwanted conduct of a sexual nature.

What to document
• Specific behavior of the offender
• Incident report according to your facility's policy

Suggested references

American Hospital Association. "HIPAA Privacy Regulations: Overview," 2015. Available: http://www.aha.org/content/00-10/overview0302.pdf.

Lockhart, L. "Sexual harassment in the workplace." *Nursing Made Incredibly Easy!* 14(6):55-55, November/December 2016. Available: http://www.nursingcenter .com/journalarticle?Article_ID=3813131&Journal_ID=417221&Issue_ID =3812948.

Nebraska Hospital Association. "Guide to HIPAA Compliance in News and Media Relations," 2015. Available: www.nebraskahospitals.org/file_download /8be9e2dd-e18e-412c-a6c8-84364c97de02.

Radoslovich, N. "Bullying in the Health Care Environment," *Plastic Surgical Nursing* 34(2):70-71, April-June 2014. Available: http://www.nursingcenter.com /journalarticle?Article_ID=2483458&Journal_ID=496448&Issue_ID=2483345.

Smith, L. "Chart Smart: Documenting with Photographs," *Nursing* 37(8):20-20, 2018. Available: http://www.nursingcenter.com/journalarticle?Article _ID=734590&Journal_ID=54016&Issue_ID=734568.

The Joint Commission. "Bullying Has No Place in Healthcare," *Quick Safety* (24), June 2016. Available: https://www.jointcommission.org/issues/article.aspx?Article =rFhOFvmOhideyaeaXWHwdF7iIsdGP TcEobEhA7d2RU=.

U.S. Department of Health & Human Services. "Summary of HIPAA Privacy Rule," 2013. Available: https://www.hhs.gov/hipaa/for-professionals/privacy/laws -regulations/index.html.

Chapter 9

Acute care documentation

Just the facts

In this chapter, you'll learn:

♦ medical record forms used in acute care settings

♦ contents and organization of those forms

♦ advantages and disadvantages of each form

♦ more detailed information about care pathways.

A look at acute care

A recent study found that most documentation efforts fail to meet legal and professional standards when examined—this is in sharp contrast to the many care providers who believe that their documentation is "good" or "adequate."

Are you one of them? Like many nurses working in acute care settings, you may feel discouraged—even overwhelmed—by the amount of information you have to document each day. You may also be baffled by some methods of documentation, such as computerized documentation, flow sheets, and care pathway. Ironically, formats that are meant to save time for nurses may actually end up costing time. Nurses accustomed to writing long, handwritten notes may be uncomfortable taking advantage of shortcuts offered by newer methods, especially given today's litigious environment, in which documentation is strongly linked to liability. The result: Many nurses end up double documenting—for example, recording the information with a check mark on a flow sheet and then documenting it again in longhand in progress notes.

Evidence shows that accurate documentation improves clinical outcomes, processes of care, and professional practice. Let's start improving your nursing documentation by examining some of the barriers that impact quality documentation. Knowing the barriers can be the first step in breaking them down!

Barriers to documentation

With the increase in multisystem diseases in our patient population and the challenge of new care innovations, confusion over what to document is a common complaint. This, along with too many documentation requirements, is often cited as a reason nurses feel that they can't spend enough time with their patients. Some estimates are that nurses in acute care can spend up to 50% of their time documenting! However, in the long run, taking the time to carefully commit patient information to the medical record in a timely fashion frees you to spend more time on direct patient care.

Additionally, two of the most frequent allegations against nurses in medical liability claims relates to the timing of documentation and the absence of documentation when it should exist. (See *Didn't document, didn't do.*)

To break down these barriers, your best weapon is familiarity. There are many formats of nursing documentation available, but none is the "perfect" system; each has its own advantages and disadvantages.

Case in point

Didn't document, didn't do

In the case of *Pommier v. ABC Insurance Company* (1998), a 55-year-old patient with a fractured hip underwent surgery. During surgery, the patient was immobilized on the operating table. The operating room nurse noted that the patient was able to move her toes on both feet. The day after surgery, a nurse noted that the patient had good color, motion, and strength in both feet. However, while performing rounds, the practitioner discovered that the patient had peroneal palsy in her left foot and leg. At the time of discharge, the patient was fitted with a left drop foot brace because of the condition.

The testimony

The patient and her family testified that immediately after the surgery, the patient experienced significant pain in her left leg. The nurse's notes, however, didn't contain documentation of the patient's pain.

The verdict

Ultimately, the circulating nurse and other members of the surgical team were held responsible for failing to use proper padding during surgery and for failing to document the final position check of the patient. The nurse testified that it wasn't her usual practice to document all padding used during surgery and that she always used padding around the knee in such a surgery. However, given the inability to explain another reason for the injury, the nurse's failure to document the use of padding allowed for the jury to determine that proper padding wasn't used.

Learn about them and choose the one that best suits your nursing practice. If your employer uses a particular system, learn it well and use it to its best advantage.

When documenting, make sure that your notes are of high-quality by remembering these characteristics. Nursing documentation should be fact-based and patient-focused, reflecting nursing interventions. Documentation should also be timely, sequential, nonduplicative and records variances in care.

Document care that has been given and the outcomes of that care, rather than opinions or lengthy descriptions of interventions and their rationale. As much as possible, try to document at the time that care is given. Although late entries are acceptable in certain circumstances (such as deterioration of condition in another patient on the unit), they are often seen as questionable. When necessary, document a late entry as soon as possible, and always note the reason for the lateness. Avoid saving your documentation till the end of the shift when fatigue can cause forgetfulness and lead to incomplete or inaccurate documentation. Being too busy or too tired can *never* be an excuse for poor documentation.

Is this ALWAYS the case?

Charting by exception is a method of documentation designed to minimize documentation. In this format, a notation is made only when there is a deviation from the baseline or expected outcome or when a procedure or expected activity is to be omitted. Well-defined standards of nursing care and documentation guidelines must be in place to use charting by exception effectively. Also, use the nursing process and think critically to determine if the patient's findings are normal or are exceptions to normal. When in doubt about whether an observation should be documented, err on the side of caution and document.

Computerized documentation: The electronic health record

In recent years, technology has been used more and more often in nursing documentation. The electronic health record (EHR) can focus and guide proper documentation, reduce inefficiencies, decrease errors, and ease information transfer across providers. Especially if computers are at the bedside, nursing time in direct patient care may also increase. Computers increase legibility of the record and decrease the use of abbreviations. Each entry and review is time–date stamped, protecting the patient's privacy.

However, even well-designed, computerized documentation can lead to errors. For example, the wrong item may be entered from a drop-down menus. If the system allows the "autofilling" of data from previous entries, or the ability to cut and paste, incorrectly entered information may be inadvertently repeated over and over again in the record. Poorly integrated records can lead to repetition of data in many fields—causing duplicative records. Additionally, many nurses have limited computer expertise, and if the system is complicated, time spent documenting can increase significantly. Finally, poorly functioning or not enough equipment increases staff frustration and wastes time.

Forms, forms, and more forms

Sometimes, the amount of documentation forms can be overwhelming. A medical record with well-organized, completed forms serves three purposes:

1. It helps you communicate patient information to other members of the health care team.
2. It protects you and your employer legally by providing evidence of the nature and quality of care the patient received. (See *Didn't document, didn't do*, page 207.)
3. It's used by your facility to obtain accreditation and reimbursement for care.

Although not an exhaustive list, the following forms—most commonly used to create medical records in acute care settings—are explained in this chapter:

- admission database or admission assessment forms
- nursing care plans
- care pathways
- patient care Kardexes
- graphic forms
- progress notes
- flow sheets
- discharge summary and patient discharge instruction forms.

Other forms include patient-teaching documents, dictated documentation, and patient self-documentation. New forms and formats of documentation are continually being developed.

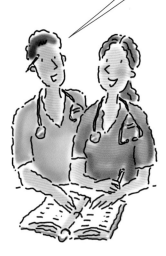

I'd hate to have to document all this information twice. That's what can happen when nurses are uncomfortable with newer methods of documentation.

Admission database form

The admission database form is used to document your initial patient assessment. The scope of information documented at this stage is usually broad, establishing a detailed baseline of clinical information against which you will compare ongoing assessments and with which you will plan the patient's care.

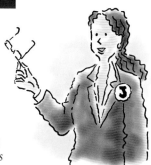

The clock is ticking

The Joint Commission requires that the admission assessment—including a health history and physical examination—be completed within 24 hours of admission; some facilities require a shorter time frame. To complete the admission database form, you must collect relevant information from various sources and analyze it. The finished form portrays a complete picture of the patient at admission.

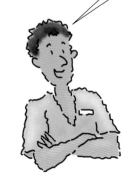

I feel like a million bucks! The wealth of information I gather during admission is invaluable.

Finding form

The admission database form may be organized in different ways. Some facilities use a form organized by body system. Others use a format that groups information to reflect such principles of nursing practice as patient response patterns.

Get it together!

More and more facilities are using integrated admission database forms. On integrated admission database forms, nursing and medical assessments complement each other, reducing the need for repeated documentation. (See *Integrated admission database form*, pages 211 to 214.)

Documentation with style

Regardless of how the form is organized, findings are documented in two basic styles:
1. standardized, open-ended style, which comes with preprinted headings and questions
2. standardized, closed-ended style, which has preprinted headings, checklists, and questions with specific responses (you simply check off the appropriate response). Most facilities use a combination of styles in one form.

As you complete the admission database form, keep in mind that the information you document is used by The Joint Commission, quality improvement groups, and other parties to continue accreditation, justify requests for reimbursement, and maintain or improve patient care standards.

Form and function

A carefully completed admission database form is extremely valuable as a description of the patient's baseline. In addition, it contains physiologic, psychosocial, and cultural information that's useful throughout the patient's stay in your facility. As such it provides:
- a holistic overview of the patient's actual and potential health problems and expectations for treatment
- insight into the patient's ability to comply with therapy and expectations for treatments
- details about the patient's lifestyle, support systems, and cultural influences that can affect how care is provided and will help in discharge planning.

(Text continues on page 215.)

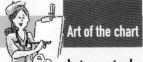

Art of the chart

Integrated admission database form

Most health care facilities use a multidisciplinary admission form. The sample form below has spaces that can be filled in by the nurse, the practitioner, and other health care providers.

Perry, Beatrice
Acct # G3058417750
ADM: 02/27/17
DOB: 01/19/66
DOWNTOWN MED CTR

Address _____2 clayton street_____
_____Dallas, Texas 55532_____
Admission Date _2_ / _27_ / _2017_ Time _1345_
Admitted per: ____ Ambulatory
✔ Stretcher ____ Wheelchair
T _98_ P _92_ R _24_ BP _98_/_52_
Ht. _5'2"_ Wt. _225 lb_
(estimated/actual)

SECTION COMPLETED BY: _____K. Crawford, CCST_____

ORIENTATION TO ROOM/UNIT POLICIES EXPLAINED

✔ Call light	____ Living will on chart
✔ Bed oper.	____ Valuables for
✔ Phone	✔ Elec.
✔ Television	✔ Smoking
✔ Meals	____ Side rails
____ Advance directive explained	✔ ID bracelet on
____ Living will	____ Visiting hours

> Be time-efficient by asking technicians or nursing assistants to get some information, if your policy allows.

TIME: _1350_

Name and phone numbers of two people to call if necessary:

NAME	RELATIONSHIP	PHONE #
Mary Ryan	daughter	665-2190
John Carr	son	665-4785

REASON FOR HOSPITALIZATION __(patient quote:) I go numb in my ℞ arm and leg__
ANTICIPATED DATE OF DISCHARGE: _____3/2/2017_____
PREVIOUS HOSPITALIZATIONS: SURGERY/ILLNESS   DATE
_____TIA_____   11/4/2015

HEALTH PROBLEM	YES	NO	?
Arthritis		✔	
Blood problem (anemia, sickle cell, clotting, bleeding)		✔	
Cancer		✔	
Diabetes	✔		
Eye problems (cataracts, glaucoma)		✔	
Heart problem		✔	
Liver problem		✔	
Hiatal hernia		✔	
High blood pressure	✔		
HIV/AIDS		✔	
Kidney problem		✔	
Comments:			

HEALTH PROBLEM	YES	NO	?
Lung problem (Emphysema, Asthma, Bronchitis, TB, Pneumonia, Shortness of breath)	✔		
Stroke		✔	
Ulcers		✔	
Thyroid problem		✔	
Psychological disorder		✔	
Alcohol abuse		✔	
Drug abuse			
Drug(s) _____			
_____		✔	
Smoking	✔		
Other _____			

ALLERGIES: ☐ TAPE ☐ IODINE ☐ LATEX ☐ no known allergies
☐ FOOD: _____   ☑ DRUG: _Penicillin_
☐ BLOOD REACTION: _____   ☐ OTHER: _____

MEDICATIONS: _____
HERBAL PREPARATIONS: _____
INFORMATION RECEIVED FROM: **SECTION COMPLETED BY:**
☑ Patient ☐ Relative _____ ☐ Friend _____ ☐ Other _____ _N. O'Meara, RN_ Date _2/27/2017_ Time _1405_

(continued)

Integrated admission database form *(continued)*

All assessment sections are to be completed by a professional nurse.   Date __2/27/2017__

> This diagram allows you to map any impairment in skin integrity.

GENERAL PHYSICAL APPEARANCE

__✓__ Clean   _____ Disheveled

SKIN INTEGRITY: Indicate the location of any of the following on the chart to the right using the designated letter: a = rashes, b = lesions, c = significant bruises/abrasions, d = burns, e = pressure sores, f = recent scars, g = presence of tubes/appliances, h = other _____

Comments: ___b: ischemic leg ulcer (2cm=healing)___

PRESSURE SORE POTENTIAL ASSESSMENT

PARAMETERS	0	1	2	3	Score
Mental status	(Alert)	Lethargic	Semicomatose	Comatose	0
			Count These Conditions As Double		
Activity	Ambulatory	(Needs help)	Chairfast	Bedfast	1
Mobility	Full	(Limited)	Very limited	Immobile	1
Incontinence	(None)	Occasional	Usually of urine	Total of urine and feces	0
Oral nutrition intake	Good	(Fair)	Poor	None	1
Oral fluid intake	(Good)	Fair	Poor	None	0
Predisposing diseases (diabetes, neuropathies, vascular disease, anemias)	Absent	Slight	Moderate	(Severe)	6
Patients with scores of 10 or above should be considered at risk.				Total	9

FALL-RISK ASSESSMENT

Impaired: ____ sensory function   ____ general debility/weakness
    ____ urinary/GI function   __✓__ history of recent falls/dizziness/blackouts
    ____ mobility function   (automatically designates patient as prone-to-fall)
    ____ mental status   __✓__ prone-to-fall risk (indicated on nursing Kardex __✓__)

NEUROLOGICAL

____ Dizziness   ____ Syncope   ____ Headache   ____ Blurred vision
____ Recent seizure   __✓__ Numbness/tingling location: ___Ⓡarm and leg___

LOC: __✓__ Alert   ____ Lethargic   ____ Semicomatose   ____ Comatose
Mental Status: __✓__ Oriented   ____ Confused   ____ Disoriented
Speech: __✓__ Clear   ____ Slurred   ____ Garbled   ____ Aphasic

Neurological Checklist

Right Arm	Right Leg	Right Pupil		Coma Scale			
Left Arm	Left Leg	Left Pupil	Pupil Reaction	Eyes Open	Best Verbal Response	Best Motor Response	Total
+2/+4	+2/+4	5/6	+	4	5	6	15

	Response	1	2	3	4	5	6
COMA SCALE CODE	EYES OPEN	Never	To Pain	To Sound	Sponta neously		
	VERBAL	None	Incomprehensible Sounds	Inappropriate words	Confused Conversation	Oriented	
	MOTOR	None	Extension	Flexion Abnormal	Flexion Withdrawal	Localizes Pain	

+1:cannot move   +3:move against gravity
+2:cannot move against gravity   +4:move strongly against gravity

Comments: ___numbness transient___

Extremities movement/strength
Pupil Reaction
- Reactive
- Nonreactive
D Dilated
C Constricted
> Greater than
< Less than
= Equal
= Sluggish

CODE
Pupils: mm
1 ·
2 ●
3 ●
4 ●
5 ●
6 ⬤
7 ⬤
8 ⬤

> These circles will help you document pupil reaction accurately.

BEHAVIORAL

Behavior: __✓__ Cooperative   ____ Uncooperative   ____ Depressed
    ____ Restless   ____ Other
    ____ Combative   __✓__ Anxious   ____ Unresponsive

Comments: _____
Religious/Spiritual beliefs: ___Lutheran___
P. request to contact minister/priest/rabbi? __✓__ Y ____ N
Name ___Reverend Thomas Jones___ Phone # ___5̶5-4792___

PAIN

Pt. having pain at present? ____ Y __✓__ N
Pt. had pain in last several months? ____ Y __✓__ N
Rate pain on a scale of 0–10 (0 = no pain, 10 = severe pain) _____
Pain location _____ Quality _____

Radiation ____ Y ____ N Duration _____
What aggravates pain? _____ What alleviates ____?
Effects on ADLs _____
Pt. pain goals _____

Integrated admission database form *(continued)*

| Addressograph | Date _2/27/2017_ |

CARDIOVASCULAR

Skin Color: ____ Normal ____ Flushed ____ Pale __✓__ Cyanotic
Apical Pulse: ____ Regular __✓__ Irregular ____ Pacemaker: Type ____   Rate ____
Peripheral Pulses: __✓__ Present ____ Equal __✓__ Weak ____ Absent   Comments: _bilat. weak lower extremities_
Specify: R ____ radial ____ pedal   L ____ radial ____ pedal
Comments: _____
Edema: ____ No __✓__ Yes _+1 bilat. pretibial_   Numbness: ____ No __✓__ Yes   Site: _Rt. arm and leg_
Chest Pain: __✓__ No ____ Yes ____   P _____   Q _____   R _____   S _____   T _____
Family Cardiac History: ____ No __✓__ Yes   Telemetry Monitor: ____ No __✓__ Yes   rhythm _normal sinus_
Comments: _____

PULMONARY

Respirations: __✓__ Regular ____ Irregular ____ Shortness of breath ____ Dyspnea on exertion
O₂ use at home? ____ Yes __✓__ No
Chest expansion: __✓__ Symmetrical ____ Asymmetrical (explain: _____)
Breath sounds: ____ Clear ____ Crackles ____ Rhonchi __✓__ Wheezing   Location _bilat upper lobe, inspiratory_
Cough: None ____ Nonproductive ____ Productive ____ Describe _____
Comments: _pulse oximetry 98% on 2 L; sleeps with 2 pillows_

GASTROINTESTINAL

Stool: __✓__ Formed
____ Loose
____ Liquid
____ Mucus
____ Ostomy
____ Incontinent
Color: __✓__ Brown
____ Black
____ Red tinged
____ Bloody

Diarrhea ____
Constipation ____
Abdomen: __✓__ Soft
____ Rigid
____ Nontender
____ Tender
____ (Location)
Bowel Sounds __✓__ Present
____ Absent
____ Hypoactive
____ Hyperactive

Obese __✓__
thin ____
emaciated ____
nourished ____

*NUTRITION:
__✓__ Special Diet
1800 ADA
____ Tube feeding
____ Chewing problem
____ Chewing problem
____ Swallowing problems
____ Nausea/vomiting
____ Poor appetite
____ Wt. loss/gain ____ lb
* Refer to dietitian if any ✓

GENITOURINARY/REPRODUCTIVE

Color of Urine: __✓__ Yellow ____ Amber ____ Pink/Red tinged ____ Brown ____ Orange ____ Clear ____ Cloudy
____ Ileo-Conduit ____ Incontinent ____ Catheter in place ____ Frequency ____ Urgency
____ Difficulty in initiating stream ____ Pain ____ Burning ____ Oliguria ____ Anuria
____ Dialysis   Access site: _____   Date of last dialysis: _____
Comments: _____
Date of LMP _1977_ _____   Date of last PAP _5/01_ _____   Breast self-exam ____ Yes __✓__ No
Use of contraceptives: ____ Yes (type _____)   ____ No __✓__ N/A
Vaginal Discharge: ____ Yes (describe _____)   __✓__ No
Bleeding: ____ Yes (amount _____)   __✓__ No
Pregnancies: Pregnant ____ Yes ____ Weeks gravida ____ Para   __✓__ No
Date of last Prostate Exam _____   Testicular self-exam ____ Yes ____ No
Comments: _____

ACTIVITY/MOBILITY PATTERNS

____ Ambulates independently ____ Full ROM ____ Limited ROM (explain: _____)
__✓__ Ambulates with assistance (explain: _____) __✓__ cane ____ walker ____ crutches
____ Gait steady/unsteady ____ Mobility in bed (ability to turn self) ____
Musculoskeletal ____ Pain ____ Weakness ____ Contractures ____ Joint swelling
____ Paralysis ____ Deformity ____ Joint stiffness ____ Cast ____ Amputation
Describe: _____
Comments: _____

> Note that the form contains room for additional comments.

REST/SLEEP PATTERNS

____ Use of sleeping aids _____   Sleeps _6_ hr/day
Comments: _____

Additional assessment comment: _On arrival, diaphoretic with hand tremors. Vital signs stable, glucose 56 mg/dl._
Orange juice and lunch given to pt. 2 hr post prandial glucose 204. Symptoms subsided with juice.
Nutritionist and diabetes educator consulted. _____ _N. O'Meara, R.N_

(continued)

Integrated admission database form *(continued)*

EDUCATION/DISCHARGE SECTION
Instructions: Assessment sections must be completed
within 8 hours of admission. Discharge planning and summary
must be completed by day of discharge.

Addressograph

> This final page deals with patient teaching and discharge planning.

EDUCATIONAL ASSESSMENT

Yes	No	
✓		Patient understands current diagnosis
✓		Family/significant other understands diagnosis
✓		Patient able to read English
✓		Patient able to write English
✓		Patient able to communicate
	✓	Patient/family understands prehospital medication/treatment regimen

Yes	No	**Emotional Factors:**
✓		Patient appears to be co...
✓		Family appears to be cop...
	✓	Any suspicion of family v...ence
	✓	Any suspicion of family abuse
	✓	Any suspicion of family neglect

Comment: _diabetes teaching_

Language spoken, written, and read (other than English): _____
Interpreter services needed: ✓ No ___ Yes
Are there any barriers to learning (e.g., emotional, physical, cognitive)? _No_
Religious or cultural practices that may alter care or teaching needs? ___ Yes ✓ No   Describe: _____
Is pt/family motivated to learn? ✓ Yes ___ No   describe: _____

DISCHARGE ASSESSMENT

Living arrangements/caregiver (relationship): _lives alone_
Type of dwelling: ___ Apartment ✓ House ___ Nursing Home ___ More than 1 floor? ✓ Yes ___ No   Describe: _____
___ Boarding Home ___ Other _____
Physical barriers in home: ✓ No ___ Yes (explain: _____
Access to follow-up medical care: ✓ Yes ___ No (explain: _____
Ability to carry out ADL: ___ Self-care ✓ Partial assistance ___ Total assistance
Needs help with: ✓ Bathing ___ Feeding ___ Ambulation ___ Other _____
Anticipated discharge destination: ___ Home ___ Rehab. ✓ Nursing Home ___ SNF ___ Boarding Home
___ Other _____
Currently receiving services from a community agency? ___ Yes ___ No
If yes, check which one ___ visiting nurses ___ Meals on Wheels
Concerned about returning home? ___ Being alone ___ Financial problems ___ Homemaking ___ Meal prep.
___ Managing ADLs ___ Other _____
Assessment completed by: _N. O'Meara, RN_   Date _2/27/2017_   Time _1430_

> This assessment form is multidisciplinary. In this example, nurses and doctors provided information.

DISCHARGE PLANNING

Resources notified:	Name	Date	Time	Signature
Social worker				
Home care coordinator	M. Murphy, RN	2/28/2017	0900	M. Murphy, RN
Other _____				

Equipment/Supplies needed: _stair chair_
Arranged for by: _M. Murphy, RN_   Date _2/28/2017_   Time _0930_
Comment: _daughter to stay with pt at home_

DISCHARGE SUMMARY

Alterations in patterns: If yes, explain.	Yes	No	Explanation
Nutrition	✓		adherence to ADA diet regimen
Elimination		✓	
Self-care		✓	
Skin integrity		✓	
Mobility	✓		needs help with stairs
Comfort pain		✓	
Mental status/behavior		✓	
Vision/Hearing/Speech		✓	

Discharge instructions given (specify): _standard hosp. discharge instruction sheet_
Effects of illness on employment/lifestyle: _____
Central venous line removed: _N/A_   By whom: _____
Belongings sent with patient: ✓ clothes ✓ dentures ✓ eyeglasses ___ hearing aid ___ prosthesis ___ valuables
✓ prescriptions ✓ other _cane_
Follow-up medical supervision to be provided by: _Dr. W. Schran_
✓ Patient/family instructed to call for follow-up appointment   Discharge destination: _pt's home with daughter_
Section completed by: _C. Rafferty, RN_   Date _3/2/2017_   Time _12/5_

How to use the admission database form

Conduct the patient interview and record the information on the admission form or progress notes as soon as possible, noting the date and time of the entry.

In some cases, you can ask the patient to complete a questionnaire about past and present health status and use this to document health history.

Ready, willing, and able?

Before completing the admission database form, try to create a private environment and consider the patient's ability and readiness to participate. For example, if the patient is sedated, confused, hostile, angry, or having pain or breathing problems, ask only the most essential questions. You can perform an in-depth interview later, when the patient's condition improves.

Turning to friends and family

If the patient can't provide information, consider seeking help from friends or family members. Be sure to document your sources. If neither the patient nor the family is able to participate, base your initial assessment on your observations and physical examination.

Too many cooks . . . er, health care workers . . . can spoil the chart

Many other people will document on the integrated admission database forms, increasing the risk of duplicative, incorrect, or contraindicatory information. Never assume that colleagues collected the right information—review, verify, and correct information gathered by nursing assistants and licensed practical nurses practitioner.

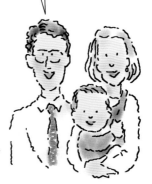

Don't forget that we can also be a source of information.

Medication reconciliation

As part of the admission process, medication reconciliation *must* occur. In this essential process, all medications that the patient is using at the time of admission (including over the counter meds and nutritional supplements) are recorded. This can be difficult if the patient doesn't remember medications or is unable to participate in the process due to medical condition. Encourage family members to bring in medication bottles from the patient's home or to provide the name of pharmacy so that the most updated list possible may be obtained.

Most facilities utilize a standardized medication reconciliation form which has spaces to enter the name, dose, route, and frequency of each medication taken. This completed list is later reviewed by the practitioner. This ensures that all essential medications are ordered for the inpatient stay, and that interactions and duplications with inpatient medications are avoided. At the time of transfer between units or facilities, medication reconciliation is performed and documented. At the time of discharge, medication reconciliation is performed, documented, and a copy is given to the patient/family and medical provider to ensure continuity of care in the outpatient setting.

Care plans and care pathways

In acute care settings today, two different formats are being used to guide the process of care for a patient:
1. traditional care plan
2. care pathway.

Both formats offer important advantages and disadvantages; sometimes they are even used together to obtain the advantages of both.

Care plans

The traditional care plan, based on the nursing process, is a tool that is used among the nurses on the patient's case. Focused in this way, the care plan provides a precise account of the patient's individual diagnoses, nursing needs, and the plan to address them. (See *Care plan requirements.*) (For more information on care plans, see chapter 3, Care plans.)

Care pathways

The care pathway (also called a *critical pathway*) is a tool developed by nurses, practitioners, and other health care providers for a specific diagnosis-related group (DRG). The pathway outlines a patient's daily care requirements and desired outcomes for routine conditions.

Care pathways work best with diagnoses that have fairly predictable outcomes—for example, hip replacement, stroke, myocardial infarction, and open heart surgery. Often, a case manager oversees the achievement of outcomes, length of stay, and the use of resources throughout the patient's illness. Pathways help to ensure that patients receive quality care in a most cost-effective manner.

Watch your step on the pathway

Using a care pathway doesn't eliminate the need for nurses to diagnose and treat human responses to health problems. Patients are individuals and commonly require nursing intervention beyond that specified in the care pathway.

For example, a patient enters the hospital for a hip replacement and can't communicate verbally because of a previous stroke. The care pathway wouldn't include measures to assist this patient in making personal needs known. Therefore, you would develop a nursing care

Care plan requirements

Although The Joint Commission no longer requires a specific care-planning format, it does require that this information be included in care plans in an acute care setting:
• ongoing assessments of the patient's illness, needs, concerns, problems, capabilities, and limitations
• notation of nursing interventions and patient responses to care
• ongoing evaluation and modification of nursing diagnoses, interventions, and expected outcomes
• reevaluation of patient progress compared to goals of the care plan
• documentation of the inability to meet patient care goals and the reasons.

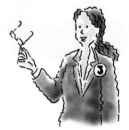

plan around the nursing diagnosis *Impaired verbal communication.* By using the diagnosis-based care pathway and modifying it based on the patient's individual nursing diagnoses, you can provide the best in collaborative care to meet the patient's specific needs. (For more information about care pathways, see chapter 3, Care plans.)

Patient care Kardex

The patient care Kardex, sometimes called the *nursing Kardex*, gives a quick overview of basic patient care information.   A Kardex can be computer-generated, or it may be a checklist format, on which the nurse can mark off items that apply to the patient. It also contains space for recording current orders for medications, patient care activities, treatments, and tests. (See *Considering the Kardex*, pages 218 and 219.)

A Kardex isn't a Joint Commission requirement. Some facilities have eliminated the use of Kardexes, incorporating the information they contain into the patient's care plan.

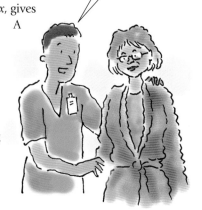

Critical pathways have their advantages, but you still must address your patient's individual needs.

It's all in the Kardex

Refer to the Kardex during change-of-shift reports and update it throughout the day. The information it contains usually includes:
- patient's name, age, marital status, and religion
- medical diagnoses, listed by priority
- nursing diagnoses, listed by priority
- results of diagnostic tests and procedures, vital signs, intake and output
- current practitioners' orders for medication, treatments, diet, intravenous (I.V.) therapy, diagnostic tests, procedures, and consultations.

The Kardex can be all aces

The Kardex has some good points, including:
- It allows quick access to information about task-oriented interventions, such as medication administration and ancillary testing and teaching.
- It records information that helps nurses plan daily interventions, such as the time a patient prefers to bathe, food preferences, and which analgesics or positions are usually required to ease pain.
- It can be used in and tailored to the needs of a particular setting.
- The care plan may be added to the Kardex to provide all the necessary data for patient care, although this can duplicate information.

(Text continues on page 220.)

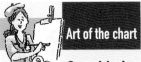

Art of the chart

Considering the Kardex

Here's an example of a patient care Kardex for a critical care unit. Remember that the categories, words, and phrases on a Kardex are brief and intended to trigger images of special circumstances, procedures, activities, or patient conditions.

Care status
Self-care ☐
Partial care with assistance ☐
Complete care ☑
Shower with assistance ☐
Tub ☐
Active exercises ☐
Passive exercises ☐

Special Care
Back care ☑
Mouth care ☑
Foot care ☐
Perineal care ☑
Catheter care ☐
Tracheostomy care ☐
Other (specify) _____ ☐

Condition
Satisfactory ☐
Fair ☐
Guarded ☑
Critical ☐
No code ☐
Advance directive?
   Yes ☑
   No ☐
Date _____3/12/2017_____

Prosthesis
Dentures
   upper ☑
   lower ☑
Contact lenses ☐
Glasses ☑
Hearing aid ☑
Other (specify) _____ ☐

Isolation
Strict ☐
Contact ☐
Airborne ☑
Neutropenic ☐
Droplet ☐
Other (specify) _____ ☐

Diet
Type: _low-fat, no conc. sweets_
Force fluids ☐
NPO ☐
Assist with feeding ☐
Isolation tray ☑
Calorie count ☐
Supplements _____

Tube feedings ☐
Type: _____
Rate: _____
Route: _____
   NG ☐
   G tube ☐
   J tube ☐

Admission
Height: _60"_
Weight: _145 lb (65.8 kg)_
BP: _124/72_
TPR: _100.4 T.P.O. - 92-24_

Frequency
BP: _q 1hr_
TPR: _q 1hr_
Apical pulses: _____
Peripheral pulses: _q 1hr_
Weight: _____
Neuro check: _____
Monitor: _____
Strips: _____
Turn: _____
Cough: _q 1hr_
Deep breathe: _q 1hr_
Central venous pressure: _____
Other (specify) _____

GI tubes
Salem sump ☐
Levin tube ☐
Feeding tube ☐
Type (specify): _____
Other (specify): _____ ☐

Activity
Bed rest ☑
Chair t.i.d. ☐
Dangle ☐
Commode ☐
Commode with assist ☐
Ambulate ☐
BRP ☐
Fall-risk category (specify): _____ ☐
Other (specify): _____ ☐

Mode of transport
Wheelchair ☐
Stretcher ☑
With oxygen ☑

I.V. devices
Saline lock ☐
Peripheral I.V. ☐
Central venous access device ☐
Triple-lumen access device ☑
Hickman ☐
Jugular ☐
Peripherally inserted ☐
PICC ☐
Parenteral nutrition ☐
Irrigations: _____

Dressings
Type: _____
Change: _CVP_
     as needed

> The check marks are intended to alert you to important patient care considerations.

Considering the Kardex *(continued)*

> You can quickly find the information you need with this format.

...apy ☐

Liters/minute _____
Method
  Nasal cannula ☐
  Face mask ☐
  Venturi (Venti) mask ☐
  Nonrebreather mask ☐
  Trach collar ☐
Nebulizer ☐
Chest PT ☐
Incentive spirometry ☐
T-piece ☐
Other (specify) _____

Drains
Type: _____
Number: _____
Location: _____

Urine Output
I&O ☑
Strain urine ☐
Indwelling catheter ☑
Date inserted _3/12/2017_
Size: _16 Fr._
Intermittent catheter ☐
  Frequency: _____

Side rails
Constant ☐
PRN ☐
Nights ☐

Restraints
Date: _____
Type: _____

Specimens and tests
CBC daily
24-hour collection
Other (specify) _____

Stools

Special notes

Social services
Consulted 3/12/2017

Monitoring
Hardwire ☑
Telemetry ☐

Pulmonary artery catheter ☑
  Pulmonary artery
  pressure _q1h_
  Pulmonary artery
  wedge pressure: _q2h_
CVP _____
Arterial line ☐
Other (specify) _ICP_ ☑

Mechanical ventilation
Type: _____
Tidal volume: _700 ml_
FIO_2 _50%_
Mode: _AC_
Rate: _12_

> On an obstetrics unit, you might find additional information on the Kardex cover sheet.

Delivery
Date: _____
Time: _____
Type of delivery: _____

Special procedures
Perineal rinse ☐
Sitz bath ☐
Witch hazel compress ☐
Breast binders ☐
Ice ☐
Abdominal binders ☐
Other (specify) _____ ☐

Mother
Due date: _____
Gravida: _____
Para: _____
Rh: _____
Blood type: _____
Membranes ruptured: _____
Episiotomy ☐
Lacerations ☐
RhoGAM studies?
  Yes ☐
  No ☐
Rubella titer?
  Yes ☐
  No ☐

Infant
Male ☐
Female ☐
Full term ☐
Premature ☐
  Weeks ☐
Apgar score ☐
Nursing ☐
Formula ☐
Condition (specify): _____
Other (specify): _____

A key Kardex kriticism

The Kardex has one major drawback: It's only as useful as nurses make it. It isn't an effective documentation tool if there isn't enough space for appropriate information, if it isn't updated frequently, if it isn't completed, or if it isn't read before giving patient care.

In addition, Kardexes aren't usually part of the permanent record, so the nurse must both update the medical record and the Kardex. Because of this, many nurses feel that updating the Kardex leads to duplicative documentation and increases the possibility of errors and contradictory entries. Computer generated Kardexes may solve this issue, as the data entered throughout the shift when providing care is later used to update the Kardex.

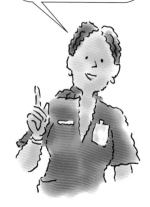

Remember: The Kardex is only as useful as you make it!

The medication Kardex

If your facility does not utilize an electronic medication administration system, it will use a medication Kardex which serves as the medication administration record (MAR). This Kardex lists the patient's ordered medications, doses, and frequency and route of administration. Medication administration is documented on this form, which is a permanent part of the patient's record. (See *The medication Kardex*, pages 221 and 222.)

Getting the most out of your medication Kardex

When recording information on a medication Kardex, here are some tips:

- After giving the first dose of a medication, sign your full name, your licensure status, and your initials in the appropriate space.
- Include the date and administration time as well as the medication dose, route, and frequency. Don't forget to initial the entry.
- Indicate when you administer a stat dose of a medication and, if appropriate, the number of doses ordered and the stop date.
- Write legibly, using only standard approved abbreviations. When in doubt about how to abbreviate a term, spell it out.
- After withholding a medication dose, document which dose wasn't given (usually by circling the time it was scheduled) and note the reason it was omitted—for example, withholding medications from a patient because of surgery scheduled that day.

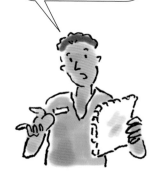

Now what does this say? I can't stress enough how important it is to write legibly!

How are things progressing? Need more space?

If you administer all medications according to the care plan, you don't need to document further. However, if your MAR doesn't have space for some information, such as the parenteral administration site, the patient's response to as-needed medications, clarifications of orders or deviations from the medication order, you'll need to record this information in the progress notes.

(Text continues on page 223.)

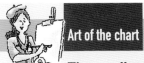

Art of the chart

The medication Kardex

One type of Kardex is the medication Kardex. It contains a permanent record of the patient's medications and may also include the patient's diagnosis and information about allergies and diet. A sample form is shown here.

NURSE'S FULL SIGNATURE, STATUS AND INITIALS	INIT.		INIT.		INIT.
Roy Charles, RN	RC				
Theresa Hopkins, RN	TH				

Don't forget to sign your name.

DIAGNOSIS: Heart failure, Atrial flutter

ALLERGIES: ASA   **DIET:** Cardiac

ROUTINE/DAILY ORDERS/FINGERSTICKS/ INSULIN COVERAGE	DATE: 3/6/2017	DATE:	DATE:	DATE:	DATE:	DATE:	DATE:	DATE:	DATE:	DATE:

ORDER DATE	MEDICATIONS DOSE, ROUTE, FREQUENCY	TIME	SITE	INT.	SITE	INT.	SITE	INT.	SITE	INT.	SITE	INT.	SITE	INT.	SITE	INT.	SITE	INT.	SITE	INT.	SITE	INT.
3/6/2017	digoxin 0.125 mg	0900	RH	RC																		
RC	I.V. daily	HR		72																		
3/6/2017	furosemide 40 mg	0900	RH	RC																		
RC	I.V. q12h	2100	RH	TH																		
3/6/2017	enalaprilat	0500	RH	TH																		
RC	1.25 mg I.V. q6h	1100	RH	RC																		
		1700	RH	RC																		

Initial in this column to verify that the dose, route, and frequency were checked against the practitioner's orders.

(continued)

The medication Kardex *(continued)*

	PRN MEDICATION				
Addressograph	ALLERGIES: ASA				

Perry, Beatrice		INITIAL	SIGNATURE & STATUS	INITIAL	SIGNATURE & STATUS
Acct # G3058417750	ADM: 03/06/17 DOB: 01/19/66 DOWNTOWN MED CTR				

YEAR 20/7   P.R.N. MEDICATIONS

ORDER DATE: 3/6/2017	RENEWAL DATE: /	DISCONTINUED DATE: /	DATE	3/6/2017									
MEDICATION: acetaminophen		DOSE 650 mg	TIME GIVEN	0930									
DIRECTION: p.r.n. pain level 1-3		ROUTE: P.O.	DATA										
			INIT.	RC									

ORDER DATE: 3/6/2017	RENEWAL DATE: 3/8/2017	DISCONTINUED DATE: /	DATE	3/6/2017									
MEDICATION: morphine sulphate		DOSE 2 mg	TIME GIVEN	1400									
DIRECTION: for pain level 4-7		ROUTE: I.V.	DATA	®A									
			INIT.	RC									

ORDER DATE: 3/6/2017	RENEWAL DATE: /	DISCONTINUED DATE: /	DATE	3/6/2017									
MEDICATION: Milk of Magnesia		DOSE 30 ml	TIME GIVEN	2115									
DIRECTION: q 6h p.r.n. constipation		ROUTE: P.O.	DATA										
			INIT.	TH									

ORDER DATE: 3/6/2017	RENEWAL DATE: /	DISCONTINUED DATE: /	DATE	3/6/2017									
MEDICATION: prochlorperazine		DOSE 5 mg	TIME GIVEN	1100	2230								
DIRECTION: q 8h p.r.n.		ROUTE: I.M.	DATA	®glut.	®glut.								
prn nausea and vomiting			INIT.	RC	TH								

> I.M. sites must be charted.

ORDER DATE: /	RENEWAL DATE: /	DISCONTINUED DATE: /	DATE										
MEDICATION:		DOSE	TIME GIVEN										
DIRECTION:		ROUTE:	DATA										
			INIT.										

ORDER DATE: /	RENEWAL DATE: /	DISCONTINUED DATE: /	DATE										
MEDICATION:		DOSE	TIME GIVEN										
DIRECTION:		ROUTE:	DATA										
			INIT.										

ORDER DATE: /	RENEWAL DATE: /	DISCONTINUED DATE: /	DATE										
MEDICATION:		DOSE	TIME GIVEN										
DIRECTION:		ROUTE:	DATA										
			INIT.										

Graphic form

The graphic form is most often used to plot data that is frequently obtained, such as the patient's vital signs. Weight, intake and output, appetite, positioning, and activity level also may be documented on the graphic form. (See *Plotting along: Using a graphic form*, page 224.)

The graphic form usually has a column of data printed on the left side of the page, times and dates written across the top, and open blocks within the side and top borders. For accuracy, check to make sure that you put data in the correct time line and that the dots you plot on the graph are large enough to be seen easily. (Connect the dots if your facility requires it.)

If a medication (e.g., an antipyretic or antihypertensive) precipitates a change in a particular vital sign, document this change in the progress notes as well as on the graphic form. Be specific about the relationship between the medication and its effect.

Advantages—in graphic terms

The graphic form has two important advantages:
- It presents information at a glance, which allows more visual comparison of data than is possible in narrative-style forms. For example, if a patient's temperature goes up or down or fluctuates over time, you can detect it much more readily on a graph than in a narrative account of the patient's temperature.
- Many different pieces of data can be presented on one form, consolidating important information, saving time and space.
- Unlicensed personnel, such as nursing assistants and technicians, are allowed to document measurements on graphic forms, saving nurses valuable time.

Disadvantages—in graphic terms

Graphic forms also have disadvantages:
- If data placed on the graph aren't accurate, legible, and complete, the form is useless. Every vital sign you take should be transcribed onto the form.
- If you use information from the graph alone, you won't get a complete picture of the patient's clinical condition. You must combine the graph with narrative documentation.

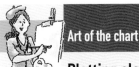

Art of the chart

Plotting along: Using a graphic form

Plotting information on a graphic form helps you visualize changes in your patient's temperature, blood pressure, heart rate, weight, and intake and output. Review the sample form below.

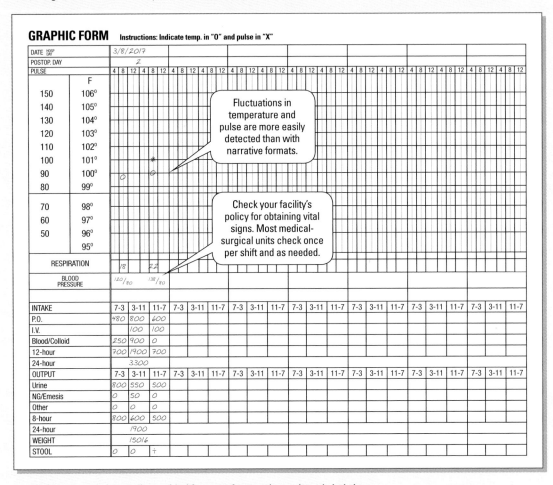

Additional space is usually provided for more frequently monitored vital signs.

DATE	TIME	BLOOD PRESSURE	PULSE	RESP.	MISCELLANEOUS
3/8/2017	0800	130/80	96	20	T 99⁴ blood transfusion
3/8/2017	0815	134/82	102	18	T 99⁸ no s/s of reaction
3/8/2017	0830	128/84	97	16	T 99²

Progress notes and flow sheets

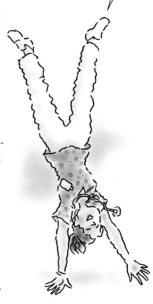

I love observing a patient's steady progress toward achieving outcomes!

In the acute care setting, progress notes and flow sheets are used to record the patient's status and monitor changes in condition. All members of the health care team can document integrated progress notes, which are in chronologic order based on the date. There are many different styles or frameworks for nursing progress notes, including narrative charting, problem-oriented approaches, and focus charting. (See chapter 4, Documentation systems.)

Regardless of the system you use, every time you write a progress note, be sure to record the exact time you gave the care or noted the observation. Note your observations of the patient's response to the care plan and if these indicate goals are or are not being met. Sometimes, nurses document a problem but fail to describe what they did as a result. If progress is not being made, document how you will change the plan of care. Avoid vague wording. Using a phrase like "appears to be" indicates uncertainty about what you're charting. Phrases like "no problems" and "had a good day" are also ambiguous. Chart specific observations instead. For example, *After repositioning and medication, patient reports his left hip has less pain, a 2 on a scale of 0 to 10. Yesterday it was a 5.*

Outline your interventions clearly, including such information as notification of other health team members, interventions, and the patient's response. For example, *Patient at 8 a.m. had oral temp of 102° F, Dr. P. Bard notified. Acetaminophen 650 mg given P.O. At 10 a.m. patient had oral temp of 100° F.*

Be sure to document new patient problems, such as onset of seizures and the resolution of old problems such as no complaint of pain in 12 hours. Also, record deteriorations in the patient's condition—for example, *Pt has increasing dyspnea, causing him to remain on bed rest. ABG values show PaO_2 of 55. O_2 provided by rebreather mask as ordered.*

All members of the health care team can document integrated progress notes, which are in chronologic order based on the date.

Making good progress

Progress notes are helpful for the following reasons:
- They're written chronologically and reflect the patient's specific nursing diagnoses. (See *Nursing diagnosis-based progress notes*, page 226.)
- They contain narrative information that doesn't easily fit into the available space or format provided by other documentation forms such as checklists.

Progress or pitfalls?

On the other hand, progress notes have these pitfalls:
- If they aren't well-organized, you may have to read through the entire form to find what you're looking for.
- You may waste time recording information on progress notes that you have already recorded on other forms and lead to duplication of the record.

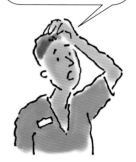

Did I already document that? I have to remember not to repeat myself.

Don't repeat yourself

Avoid including information that's already on the flow sheet, except when there's a sudden change in the patient's condition, such as a decreased level of consciousness, a change in skin condition, or swelling at an I.V. site. Together, flow sheets and progress notes usually provide adequate evidence of nursing care.

Art of the chart

Nursing diagnosis-based progress notes

Progress notes can be written using a nursing diagnosis, as the sample below shows.

Patient identification information   **Memorial General, Tempe, AZ**

Perry, Beatrice
Acct # G3058417750   ADM: 03/08/17
                      DOB: 01/19/66
MEMORIAL GENERAL
131 Green Ave.
Tempe, AZ
(123) 666-7777

Notes are directly related to the patient problem.

PROGRESS NOTES

Date and time	Nursing diagnosis and related problems	Notes
3/8/2017 – 1100	Fluid volume, excess R/T chronic renal insufficiency	Bilat. +4 pretibial and pedal edema. #16 Fr. Foley with urimeter inserted to monitor hourly output. Furosemide 40 mg I.V. given at 1055. Head of bed elevated to 45 degrees; O_2 2 L. Nasal cannula in place. ———— P.Smith, RN
3/8/2017 – 1130	Fluid volume, excess R/T chronic renal insufficiency	200 ml clear yellow urine in urimeter. Edema unchanged. Pt states: "It isn't as hard to catch my breath." — P.Smith, RN

Flow sheets

Flow sheets are used to document data related to physical assessment of the patient and record routine aspects of patient care, such as activities of daily living, fluid balance, nutrition, pain, and skin integrity. They're also useful for recording specific nursing interventions according to preestablished parameters of nursing care. documenting routine assessment data this way readily shows changes in the patient's condition and progress toward achieving expected outcomes.

The style and format of flow sheets may vary to fit the needs of patients on particular units.

Using flow sheets doesn't exempt you from narrative documentation to describe your observations, patient teaching, patient responses, detailed interventions, and unusual circumstances. (See *Let it flow*, page 228.)

Symbolic significance

Fill out flow sheets completely, using the specified symbols—such as check marks, "X"s, initials, circles, or the time—to indicate assessment of a parameter or performance of an intervention. When necessary, use the abbreviation "N/A" (not applicable) or another abbreviation recognized by your facility.

Completing the picture

Sometimes, recording only the information requested isn't enough to give a complete picture of the patient's health. In such a case, record additional information in the space provided on the flow sheet. If additional information isn't necessary, draw a line through the space to indicate this and discourage later notations. If your flow sheet doesn't have enough additional space and you need to record more information, use the progress notes. Write "see progress notes" in the space provided to indicate more in-depth data are elsewhere in the record.

Make sure that data on the flow sheet are consistent with data in your progress notes. Of course, all entries should accurately reflect the care given. Discrepancies can damage your credibility and increase your chance of liability. (See *Detail deficiency*, page 230.)

Flow sheets are easy to prepare and easy to read!

A ban on blanks

Don't leave blank spaces, which may imply that an intervention wasn't completed, wasn't attempted, or wasn't recognized. If you must omit something, document the reason for the omission. As previously noted, cross through blank spaces to note that nothing should be documented in this space.

(Text continues on page 230.)

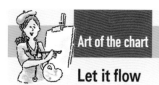

Art of the chart

Let it flow

As this sample shows, a patient care flow sheet lets you quickly document routine interventions.

PATIENT CARE FLOW SHEET

Perry, Beatrice
Acct # G3058417750
ADM: 03/08/17
DOB: 01/19/66
DOWNTOWN MED CTR

Date 3/8/2017	1900-0700	0700-1900
RESPIRATORY		
Breath sounds	Clear 1930 AS	Crackles LLL 0800 JM
Treatments/results		Nebulizer 0830 JM
Cough/results		Mod. amt. tenacious yellow mucus 0900 JM
O₂ therapy	Nasal cannula at 2 L/min AS	Nasal cannula at 2 L/min JM
CARDIAC		
Chest pain		
Heart sounds	Normal S₁ and S₂ AS	Normal S₁ and S₂ JM
Telemetry	N/A	N/A
PAIN		
Type and location	℗ flank 0400 AS	℗ flank 1000 JM
Intervention	meperidine 0415 AS	reposition and meperidine 1010 JM
Pt. response	Improved from #9 to #3 in 1/2 hour AS	Improved from #8 to #2 in 1/2 hr JM
NUTRITION		
Type		regular JM
Toleration %		90% JM
Supplement		1 can Ensure JM

Make sure that you document your patient's response to medications.

Use the flow sheet to track changes in your patient's responses.

Let it flow (continued)

PATIENT CARE FLOW SHEET

Date 3/8/2017	1900-0700	0700-1900
ELIMINATION		
Stool appearance	————————	————————
Enema	N/A	N/A
Results	————————	————————
Bowel sounds	present all quadrants 2330 AS	present all quadrants 0800 JM
Urine appearance	Clear amber 0400 AS	Clear amber 1000 JM
Indwelling urinary catheter	N/A	N/A
Catheter irrigations	————————	————————
TUBES		
Type	N/A	N/A
Irrigation	————————	————————
Drainage appearance	————————	————————
HYGIENE		
Self/partial/complete	————————	Partial 1000 JM
Oral care		1000 JM
Back care	0400 AS	1000 JM
Foot care	————————	1000 JM
Remove/reapply elastic stockings	2330 AS	1000 JM
ACTIVITY		
Type	bed rest AS	Out of bed to chair x 20 min 1000 JM
Toleration	Turns self AS	Tol. well JM
Repositioned	2330 supine AS 0400 Ⓛ side AS	Ⓛ side 0800 JM Ⓡ side 1400 JM
ROM	————————	1000 (active) JM 1400 (active) JM
SLEEP		
Sleeps well	0400 AS 0600 AS	N/A
Awake at intervals	2300 AS 0400 AS	————————
Awake most of the time	————————	————————
SAFETY		
ID bracelet on	1930 AS 0200 AS	0800 JM 1200 JM 1500 JM
Call button in reach	1930 AS 0200 AS	0800 JM 1200 JM 1500 JM
Side rails up	1930 AS 0200 AS	0800 JM 1200 JM 1500 JM

Don't leave space blank. Write "none" or "N/A" or draw a line through the space.

Flow sheets encourage you to chart care promptly.

Case in point

Detail deficiency

Thomas v. Greenview Hospital, Inc. (2004) is an example of how a lack of specific documentation can lead to legal troubles.

Patient history

An elderly patient with various medical problems, including an amputated right leg and chronic kidney disease, underwent hemiarthroplasty and remained hospitalized to receive dialysis. After surgery, the patient was considered at risk for developing pressure injuries. It was ordered that the patient be turned every 2 hours and as needed, which was consistent with the facility's written policies and procedures.

While in the facility, the patient developed a foul-smelling, stage III pressure injury that was approximately 6 3/4" × 5 7/8" (17 cm × 15 cm). Although the patient ultimately died from chronic kidney disease, the patient's family claimed that the patient developed the pressure injury as a direct result of the nursing staff's negligence and that such negligence lead to the patient's death.

Let the record speak

There were no specific entries in the patient's medical record documenting that repositioning at least every 2 hours. The nurses involved acknowledged that the chart lacked specific references to how often the patient was turned but maintained that the entries did state that safety rounds, which routinely included turning the patient, were performed every 2 hours.

The verdict

The court stated that even though there was evidence to suggest the nurses routinely turned patients as a part of their safety rounds, such evidence wasn't admissible to prove that they followed this practice when treating the patient.

Go flow sheets!

Flow sheets have many sterling qualities:

- Nursing data can be documented quickly and concisely, preferably at the time you give care or observe a change in the patient's condition.
- They allow all members of the health care team to easily compare data and assess the patient's progress over time.
- The concise format enables you to evaluate patient trends at a glance.
- They're less time-consuming to read because they tend to be more legible than handwritten progress notes.
- The format reinforces standards of nursing care and facilitates precise, less-fragmented nursing documentation.

Flow sheet faults

Flow sheets also have some less-than-ideal qualities:

- They may not have enough space for recording unusual events.
- Overuse of these forms can lead to incomplete documentation that obscures the patient's clinical picture.

- They may cause legal hassles if they aren't consistent with the progress notes. What's checked off on the flow sheet needs to agree with what's documented on the progress notes.
- The format may fail to reflect the patients' needs. Flow sheets can become a liability if they aren't tailored to each unit and revised as needed.

Discharge summaries

Discharge summaries reflect the reassessment and evaluation components of the nursing process. *To comply with The Joint Commission requirements, you must document your assessment of a patient's continuing care needs as well as any referrals for care and begin discharge planning early in the patient's stay.* The discharge process actually begins at admission when data-gathering may indicate a need for home-care, durable medical equipment, or transportation issues.

To help meet the discharge documentation requirements, many facilities combine discharge summaries and patient instructions in one form. This form contains sections for recording patient assessment and diagnostic tests findings, patient education, detailed home care instructions, or commonly-used community resource information. A discharge summary usually employs a narrative style (to tell the story of the patient's in-facility care), along with open- and closed-ended styles. (See *Moving on: Discharge summaries*, page 232.)

In sum, discharge summaries are all good

We have only good things to say about discharge summary forms:

- The combined form provides useful data about additional teaching needs and points out whether the patient has the information needed to provide personal care or to get further help.
- The form establishes compliance with The Joint Commission requirements and helps safeguard you from malpractice accusations.

How to use discharge summaries

After completing your discharge summary form, give one copy to the patient and put another copy in the medical record for future reference. Make sure that the completed form outlines the patient's care, provides useful information for further teaching and evaluation, and documents that the patient has the information needed for personal care or to get further help.

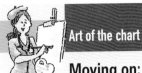

Art of the chart

Moving on: Discharge summaries

By combining the patient's discharge summary with instructions for care after discharge, you can fulfill two requirements with a single form.

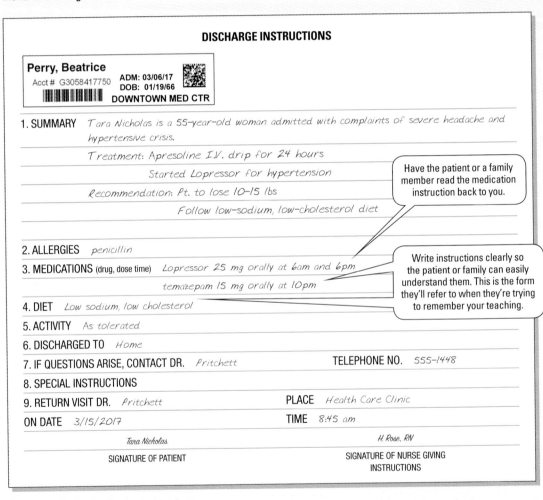

DISCHARGE INSTRUCTIONS

Perry, Beatrice
Acct # G3058417750
ADM: 03/06/17
DOB: 01/19/66
DOWNTOWN MED CTR

1. SUMMARY   *Tara Nicholas is a 55-year-old woman admitted with complaints of severe headache and hypertensive crisis.*

   Treatment: Apresoline I.V. drip for 24 hours

   Started Lopressor for hypertension

   Recommendation: Pt. to lose 10–15 lbs

   Follow low-sodium, low-cholesterol diet

> Have the patient or a family member read the medication instruction back to you.

2. ALLERGIES   *penicillin*

3. MEDICATIONS (drug, dose time)   *Lopressor 25 mg orally at 6am and 6pm*

   temazepam 15 mg orally at 10pm

> Write instructions clearly so the patient or family can easily understand them. This is the form they'll refer to when they're trying to remember your teaching.

4. DIET   *Low sodium, low cholesterol*

5. ACTIVITY   *As tolerated*

6. DISCHARGED TO   *Home*

7. IF QUESTIONS ARISE, CONTACT DR.   *Pritchett*   TELEPHONE NO.   *555-1448*

8. SPECIAL INSTRUCTIONS

9. RETURN VISIT DR.   *Pritchett*   PLACE   *Health Care Clinic*

ON DATE   *3/15/2017*   TIME   *8:45 am*

Tara Nicholas   *H. Rose, RN*

SIGNATURE OF PATIENT   SIGNATURE OF NURSE GIVING
INSTRUCTIONS

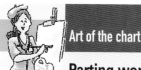

Parting words: Narrative discharge notes

Some health care facilities use a narrative-style discharge summary, which is similar to a progress note. Here's a sample.

3/9/2017	1530	Discharge summary: Pt admitted with SOB and hypertension (BP 190/100). IL nc), R/O for MI. Dx: Exac COPD. O₂ therapy administered (35% venti mask–weaned to breathing treatments initiated. Breathing improved. Pt able to participate in ADLs. Medications adjusted for BP. (BP 134/86 at 1200). Home O₂ arranged by case management. Medication reconciliation completed and reviewed with pt. Pt understands to discontinue lisinopril. Prescription for captopril 25 mg orally BID given to pt's wife, Michelle. Pt to arrange follow-up appointment with Dr. T. Harris for 10-day postdischarge appointment. Dietary changes include to follow a low-sodium diet. Activity is as tolerated. Written discharge instructions and medication reconciliation list given to pt.————— B. McCert, RN

Taking note of narrative discharge notes

Not all facilities use combined forms—some use narrative discharge notes. (See *Parting words: Narrative discharge notes.*) If your facility uses these notes, be sure to include the following information on the form:

- the patient's status at admission and discharge
- significant information about the patient's stay in the facility, including resolved and unresolved patient problems and referrals for continuing care
- instructions given to the patient, family members, and other caregivers about medications, treatments, activity, diet, referrals, follow-up appointments, and other special instructions.

Medication reconciliation

A medication reconciliation is required on admission, transfer, and discharge. By routinely reviewing the patient's home medications, errors can be avoided. At discharge, be sure to review home medications and compare to new prescriptions that the practitioner is providing or medications that the practitioner wishes the patient to discontinue. Sometimes, a duplication in medication can occur, with the patient then taking a doubled dose. Additionally, a medication may be prescribed to treat the patient, such as an antihypertensive, but the patient has a different medication at home that treats the same condition, resulting in the patient taking two medications for the same condition that may have harmful outcomes. By reconciling the patient's medication list, medications are identified that need to be continued or discontinued. This education needs to be documented as part of the discharge process.

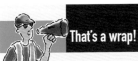

That's a wrap!

Acute care documentation review

Admission database form
- Documents patient's initial assessment
- Must be completed within 24 hours of admission
- May be integrated with nursing and medical assessments
- Contains physiologic, psychosocial, and cultural information that's used throughout hospitalization

Care plan
- Outlines the patient's nursing care
- Includes ongoing assessments, nursing diagnoses, expected outcomes, nursing interventions, and evaluation of care

Care pathway
- Is a multidisciplinary care plan that helps standardize care for routine conditions
- Determines the patient's daily care requirements and desired outcomes

Patient care Kardex
- Gives a quick overview of basic patient care information
- Allows quick access to information about task-oriented interventions, such as specific patient care, medication administration, and intravenous (I.V.) therapy
- Isn't usually a part of the permanent record, so information must also be recorded in another part of the medical record

Graphic form
- Is used to plot vital signs and other standard data
- Presents information at a glance
- Saves the nurse time because unlicensed personnel are allowed to record data on it

Progress notes
- Are used to record the patient's status and monitor the patient's condition
- Reflect the nursing process in a format that's arranged chronologically, making it easy to follow
- Allow the nurse to record information that doesn't fit into other documentation forms

Flow sheets
- Are used to record the routine aspects of care as well as specific nursing interventions, allowing you to focus on changes in the patient's condition
- Highlight specific information according to preestablished parameters of nursing care
- Commonly used to document vital signs and intake and output

Discharge summary
- Reflects the reassessment and evaluation components of the nursing process
- Commonly combined with patient discharge instruction forms
- Provides useful data about additional teaching needs and the patient's ability to care for self at home
- Establishes compliance with The Joint Commission requirements
- Contains documentation of medication reconciliation

Suggested references

Blair, W., and Smith, B. "Nursing Documentation: Frameworks and Barriers," *Contemporary Nurse* 41(2):160-168, June 2012.

College of Registered Nurses of British Columbia. "Documentation," 2017. Available: https://www.crnbc.ca/Standards/PracticeStandards/Pages/documentation.aspx.

Paans, W., et al. "Prevalence of Accurate Documentation in Patient Records," *Journal of Advanced Nursing* 66(11):2481-2489, November 2010.

RN. "Professional Nursing Documentation," 2015. Available: https://lms.rn.com/getpdf .php/2163.pdf.

Chapter 10

Home health care documentation

Just the facts

In this chapter, you'll learn:

◆ risks and responsibilities in documenting home health care

◆ forms used for home health care documentation

◆ requirements for documenting patient teaching in home health care.

A look at home health care

The purpose of home health nursing is to restore, maintain, or promote health and function for patients and their families at home. A home health agency plans, coordinates, and supplies care based on the needs of the patient and family and the resources available to them. Think of the home health agency as a hospital without walls. Home care is one component of comprehensive health care.

An emerging health care powerhouse

Trends that have contributed to the growth of the home health care industry include:

- development of a prospective payment system (PPS) for home health agencies
- use of the Outcome and Assessment Information Set (OASIS), a tool used to help assess the patient's condition
- increasing number of patients of advanced age
- increased availability of sophisticated home care equipment
- use of electronic claim processing and surveillance of the Centers for Medicare & Medicaid Services (CMS) and fiscal intermediaries.

The Balanced Budget Act of 1997 required the development of a PPS for Medicare home health services and the implementation of this system in October 2000. Under this system, Medicare pays home health agencies a predetermined base payment. The payment is adjusted for the health care needs and conditions of the patient.

Quicker has equaled sicker

Managed care organizations have identified sophisticated methods of performing utilization review, causing a decrease in the average length of stay. Therefore, patients are typically sicker when they're discharged to home.

Because support services in the home and community cost less than institutional care, government and private insurance payers have expanded their coverage of home health care.

Not your traditional patient

Traditionally, homebound Medicare recipients have constituted the major portion of the home health caseload. Agencies have expanded services to new populations, representing all age-groups and a variety of medical conditions. This expansion has led to the emergence of home health subspecialties, such as home infusion agencies and high-tech cancer-related home care, including stem cell transplants as well as home hospice services. These agencies may be offshoots of parent organizations or stand-alone agencies. (See *The hospice alternative*, page 238.)

Documentation requirements

The purpose of an OASIS assessment is to improve standardization of assessment items in post-acute care (PAC) settings. An OASIS assessment is required for all Medicare and Medicaid patients older than age 18 years, excluding women receiving maternal–child services who are receiving skilled services.

OASIS regulations require that nurses complete an initial assessment and that agencies transmit the assessment and other data within strict time frames. Not all assessment items need to be completed at every assessment.

Patient assessment must be completed:
- within 5 days of the start of care and within 5 days of the end of each 60-day recertification period
- within 48 hours after:
  - the patient is transferred to inpatient care
  - resuming care after an inpatient stay
  - the patient is discharged from home care
  - there's a significant change in the patient's condition
  - if the patient dies at home.

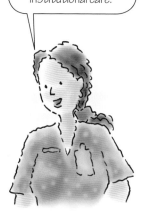

Home health services are expanding in part because they cost less than institutional care.

Creating opportunities for care

Before receiving care from a home health care agency, patients with private insurance must obtain authorization from their insurance providers. In many cases, insurance limitations restrict treatment options.

The hospice alternative

Many home health care agencies provide hospice care services. Hospice programs provide end-of-life care to terminally ill patients in both homes and hospitals.

Medicare coverage

Since 1983, patients who have met specific admission criteria can qualify for the hospice Medicare benefit instead of the traditional Medicare benefit, allowing greater freedom to choose the hospice alternative for end-of-life care. The patient receives noncurative medical and support service not otherwise covered by Medicare.

Medicare coverage for hospice care is available if:

• the patient is eligible for Medicare Part A, which covers skilled nursing home and hospital care; people eligible for Medicare include those who are age 65 years or older, long-term disabled patients, and people with end-stage renal disease.
• the patient's practitioner and the hospice medical director certify that the patient is terminally ill with a life expectancy of 6 months or less.
• the patient receives care from a Medicare-approved hospice program.

A Medicare-approved hospice program will usually provide care in the patient's home. The hospice team and the patient's practitioner establish a care plan for medical and support services for the management of a terminal illness.

A patient without coverage for hospice benefits may be eligible for free or reduced-cost care through local programs or foundations. Alternatively, a patient may pay privately for hospice services.

Understanding and acceptance of treatment

With hospice care, the patient or primary caregiver must complete documentation, indicating their understanding of hospice care. The patient or caregiver must sign an informed consent form that outlines everyone's responsibilities. The patient or primary caregiver must also sign a form indicating understanding and acceptance of the role of the primary caregiver. The form below is an example of this type of document.

REEDSVILLE HOME HEALTH AND HOSPICE
ACCEPTANCE OF PRIMARY CAREGIVER ROLE

I have been offered the opportunity to ask questions regarding the Hospice program and Hospice care of this patient. I understand that the Hospice program provides palliative, or comfort, measures and services, but not aggressive, invasive, or life-sustaining procedures.

I also understand that the Hospice concept of care is based upon the active participation of a primary care person who is not provided through the Hospice benefit, who is and will be willing to assist this patient with personal care and with activities of daily living as well as with safety precautions when Hospice personnel are not scheduled to be in the home. I accept the responsibility of being primary care-giver, and I agree to make appropriate arrangements to provide this role to this patient.

If, for any reason, I am unable to serve in this capacity at a time as deemed necessary for the safety and care of this patient, I agree to make other arrangements to fulfill the responsibilities of primary caregiver that are acceptable to Reedsville Home Health and Hospice. I further understand that Reedsville Home Health and Hospice will assist in making the arrangements but that I will be financially responsible for any costs associated with them.

Name of patient: _Joan Powell_

Signature of patient: _Joan Powell_

Date: _2/25/2017_

Name of primary caregiver: _Joseph Powell_

Date: _2/25/2017_

Signature of primary caregiver: _Joseph Powell_

Relationship: _husband_

Witness: _Cathy Melvin, RN_

Date: _2/25/2017_

> When the patient and caregiver sign this form, it indicates that they understand the purpose and goals of hospice care and agree to comply with regulations for hospice eligibility.

In this cost-conscious environment, nurses take on an especially important role in helping patients get coverage by educating them about local, state, and federal benefit programs. When you help a patient identify a needed service—such as veteran's benefits or Meals on Wheels—you can assist the patient in setting up services while ensuring that your agency receives proper reimbursement.

Legal risks and responsibilities

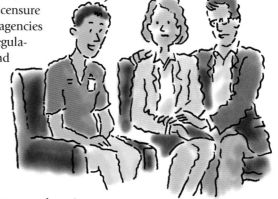

I'll help you find programs that augment your health coverage. That way, we both win.

Home health agencies are licensed and regulated by state governments and accredited by private agencies such as the Community Health Accreditation Partner (CHAP), which is administered through the National League for Nursing (NLN) and The Joint Commission. In many cases, obtaining state licensure hinges on having accreditation. Home health agencies must also adhere to Medicare and Medicaid regulations administered by CMS and its agencies and carriers.

Meeting standards

Home health agencies are evaluated for such factors as accurate and complete documentation and adherence to standards, particularly establishing eligibility for services and quality of care. If standards aren't met, a home health agency may fail to earn licensure or accreditation, may have its current license and accreditation revoked, or may have reimbursement privileges withheld or revoked.

Risks of poor documentation

Home health agencies must maintain complete and legally sound documentation. For reimbursable services, nurses must document each instance that the specified service is provided. Nurses must also document the services the agency refuses to provide. Inadequate or incomplete documentation can have serious consequences.

Evaluating admissions

Since the inception of PPS for home health agencies, agencies have had to carefully evaluate admissions. Because of this evaluation process, not all patients who are referred for home health care qualify. If a patient has no caregiver or has a complex chronic medical condition, the cost of needed care may quickly exceed the allotted reimbursement. Therefore, home health care agencies are unable to admit these patients.

Let's admit it: Admission assessment is crucial

A complete admission assessment and detailed documentation of this assessment are crucial in determining the appropriateness of each patient referred for admission.

Liability

After a nurse or home health agency is named in a lawsuit, it's too late to correct inaccurate or incomplete documentation. For example, a nurse fails to record the patient's apical pulse and rhythm before administering digoxin. Later, the family sues the home health agency, alleging the staff caused the patient to go into complete heart block by failing to recognize signs of digoxin toxicity.

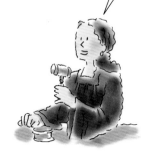

Court is in session. Let's see that record. It's too late for corrections now.

No record, no proof

Without a documented record, the agency is unable to prove that the patient wasn't experiencing excessive slowing of the pulse, a classic sign of digoxin toxicity.

Financial losses

Inadequate or incomplete documentation may result in refusal by third-party payers or fiscal intermediaries to cover services.

A bad business practice

Insurance companies who negotiate preferred provider contracts may refuse to do business with home health agencies that provide incomplete documentation.

Documentation guidelines

Documentation of care and discharge planning begins when you evaluate a new patient for service. (See *Does the patient qualify?* page 241.) You may use a referral form or specialized computer program to document the patient's needs. (See *Referral form,* pages 242 and 243.) Patients and caregivers also fill out several forms during the initial home visit. (See *Paperwork for patients,* page 241.)

Be sure to begin at the beginning

When you start caring for a patient, always document activities completed during your nursing visit: assessments, interventions, the patient's understanding and response to treatment, and whether complications occurred. Also, record your communications with family members or caregiver and other members of the health care team and the date of the next visit.

Does the patient qualify?

Careful screening, which is done at the initial evaluation, is critical when determining what clinical services a patient needs. When evaluating a new patient for service, look for the following criteria.

Clinical criteria
- Homebound status
- Skilled care needed; medically necessary
- Appropriately prescribed therapies that can be done in the home
- Ability to progress from therapies
- Caregiver available to assist patient

Technical criteria (patient or caregiver)
- Senses intact
- Ability to learn and follow procedures

- Ability to recognize complications and initiate emergency medical procedures

Environmental criteria
- Access to a telephone
- Access to electricity
- Access to water
- Clean living environment

Financial criteria
- Verification of insurance coverage
- Full knowledge of copayment or out-of-pocket expenses
- Agreement to comply with the conditions of participation

The information you provide gets around

The information you provide is used by third-party payers during utilization review to evaluate each claim in accordance with criteria for coverage. It may also be used by the government and oversight agencies to determine the validity of services.

Documentation details

Home care documentation should cover:
- OASIS information
- evidence that the home environment is safe for the procedure or treatment or can be safely adapted; findings about the home and measures taken to ensure safe delivery of care
- rationale for treatment and patient response
- *emergency and resource numbers given to the patient or caregiver (The Joint Commission requires that the patient or caregiver have 24-hour emergency telephone access to the agency or nurse.)*

(Text continues on page 244.)

Paperwork for patients

During your initial home visit, you'll ask the patient or caregiver to read and sign many forms. These required forms include:
- patient rights and responsibilities
- advance directives, including a do-not-resuscitate option
- consent for services
- medical information authorization and release
- privacy statement
- assignment of benefits
- equipment acceptance
- medication reconciliation list
- patient-teaching checklist
- emergency preparedness plan.

If an intravenous (I.V.) infusion is required, the forms also include:
- consent for vascular access
- infusion treatment service agreement.

Feeling validated
In addition, your agency may require the patient to cosign the Outcome and Assessment Information Set form and the nurses' notes or a time sheet to validate your visit in the home.

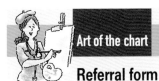

Art of the chart

Referral form

Also called an intake form, a referral form is used to document the patient's needs when you begin your evaluation of a new patient. Use the form shown here as a guide.

Date of referral: _2/26/2017_   Branch _____   ⟨This form provides an overview of the patient's condition, required treatment, and psychosocial and cultural concerns.⟩   H ✓

Info taken by: _Beth Isham, RN_   _North_   27/2017

Patient's name: _Geraldine Rush_

Address: _66 Newton St._

City: _Burlington_   State: _VT_   Zip: _05402_

Phone: _(802) 123-4567_   Date of birth: _4/3/25_

Primary caregiver name & phone number: _husband (Dennis) (802) 123-4567_

Insurance name: _Medicare_   Ins. #: _123-45-6789_

Is this a managed care policy (HMO)? _no_

Primary Dx: (Code _162.5_) _lung cancer_   Date: _2/20/2017_

(Code _811_) _pressure ulcer (coccyx)_   Date: _2/22/2017_

(Code _714.0_) _rheumatoid arthritis_   Date: _1980_

Procedure: (Code _86.28_) _pressure ulcer_   Date: _2/10/2017_

Referral source: _J. Silva, hospital SW_   Phone: _765-2813_

Doctor name & phone #: _Frank Crabbe_   Phone: _765-4321_

Doctor address: _9073 Parkway Drive, Burlington_

Hospital _University Hospital_   Admit _2/10/2017_   Discharge _2/25/2017_

Functional limitations: Pain management, _nonambulatory, poor fine motor skills due to rheumatoid arthritis_

ORDERS/SERVICES: (specify amount, frequency, and duration)

(SN:) _SN visits 3x/week & p.r.n. x 2 months_   ⟨Check out this part of the form to determine what services the patient needs.⟩

(AL:) _CNA visits 4 hours daily 5 days/week x 2 months_

(PT, OT, ST: _PT & OT evaluations and visits 2-3 x/week & p.r.n. x 2 months_

(MSW:) _MSW evaluation & weekly vs x 2 months_

Spiritual coordinator: _Rev. Carlson, St. Paul's Lutheran Church_

Counselor: _JoAnne Knowlton, MSW_

Volunteer: _Rosalie Marshall - niece will provide care on weekends_

Other services provided: _shopping, laundry, meal prep_

Goals: _wound care, pain management, terminal care at home_

Equipment: _needs: commode, hospital bed, bedpan, Hoyer lift, side rail w/c_

Company & Phone number: _Scott Medical Equipment   765-9931_

Safety Measures _side rails↑_   Nutritional req _diet as tolerated_

FUNCTIONAL LIMITATIONS: (Circle Applicable)			ACTIVITIES PERMITTED: (Circle Applicable)		
1. Amputation	5. Paralysis	9. Legally blind	1. Complete bedrest	6. Partial wgt bearing	Ⓐ Wheelchair
2. Bowel/Bladder	⑥ Endurance	A. Dyspnea with	2. Bedrest BRP	7. Independent at home	B. Walker
3. Contracture	⑦ Ambulation	minimal exer	3. Up as tolerated	8. Crutches	C. No restriction
4. Hearing	8. Speech	Ⓑ Other _R.A._	④ Transfer bed/chair	9. Cane	D. Other—specify

Accessibility to bath   Y - Ⓝ   Shower Y - Ⓝ   Bathroom Y - Ⓝ   Exit Y - Ⓝ

Mental status: (Circle) Oriented Comatose Forgetful (Depressed) Disoriented Lethargic Agitated Other

Referral form *(continued)*

Allergies: _none known_

- Hospice appropriate meds
- Med company: _Walker Pharmacy_

MEDICATIONS:

morphine sulfate liq. 20 mg/ml   40 mg P.O.   q6h p.r.n. pain

Reglan 10 mg P.O. q.i.d. p.r.n. nausea/vomiting

Colace 200 mg P.O. daily p.r.n. constipation

Benadryl 25–50 mg P.O. at bedtime p.r.n. sleeplessness

Living will   yes _✓_   no _____   obtained _____   Family to mail to office _____

Guardian, POA, or responsible person: _husband_

Address & phone number: _same_

Other family members: _____

ETOH _0_   Drug Use: _0_   Smoker _2 ppd x 40 years quit 2 yrs ago_

History: _Other than problems associated with arthritis, was in general good health until 12/07. Dx: lung CA – husband_ _cared for at home until 11/08._

Social history (place of birth, education, jobs, retirement, etc.): _Born & raised in Toronto, became U.S. citizen_ _when married in 1951. 2 yrs. college – majored in music. Retired church organist._

ADMISSION NOTES: VS: T _98° P.O._   AP _86_   RR _18_   BP _140/72_

Lungs: _decreased breath sounds LLL._   Extremities: _cool to touch Pedal pulses present._

Wgt _118_   Recent wgt/loss/gain of _40 lb over 6 months_

Admission narrative: _visit made to pt/husband in hospital before discharge. Both have been told that she is failing_ _rapidly, and would like her to return home with Hospice services. Niece willing to help 2 days/week. Pt apprehensive;_ _husband blames himself for the coccygeal decubitus that developed under his care._

Psychosocial issues: _Pt has always cared for husband. Describes self as depressed that she is no longer able to do_ _so; worries who will care for him after she dies._

Environmental concerns: _(need smoke detectors)_

Are there any cultural or spiritual customs or beliefs of which we should be aware before providing Hospice services? _Pt would like Holy Communion just before death (& weekly)_

Funeral home: _not yet chosen_   Contact made? yes _____   no _x_

DIRECTIONS: _corner Newton / Elm duplex, white with green trim. Door on (L) says 66. Bell broken – knock loudly._

Agency Representative Signature: _Beth Isham, RN_   Date: _2/27/2017_

Home Care Supervisor

- patient's or caregiver's ability to perform steps in home care procedures, including the ability to perform return demonstration
- patient's or caregiver's ability to troubleshoot equipment, including a backup plan for a power failure
- patient's or caregiver's ability to recognize potential complications, respond appropriately, and get help when necessary.

Home health care forms

Key information to document involving home health care includes:
- agency assessment and OASIS forms
- care plan
- progress notes
- patient-teaching sheets
- nursing and discharge summaries
- Medicare-mandated information, including home health certification and care plan, medical update, and patient information.

Agency assessment and OASIS documentation

When a patient is referred to your home health care agency, you must complete a thorough and specific assessment and document the information on a patient assessment form.

Assess the patient's:
- physical status
- functional status
- mental and emotional status
- home environment in relation to safety and support services
- knowledge of disease or current condition, prognosis, and treatment plan
- potential for complying with the treatment plan.

Guidelines for use

As with any setting, be thorough during home health care. A thorough patient assessment provides the information you need to plan appropriate care.

Consider the following guidelines:
- Obtain information about the patient's past and current health. Organize the interview by body system, and ask open-ended questions.
- When performing a physical assessment, use a systematic approach, as is appropriate in any setting. For example, you may use a body-system or head-to-toe approach.

- When assessing functional abilities, have the patient demonstrate ability in addition to answering the questions.
- When assessing the home environment, consider such factors as the presence of a caregiver, structural barriers, access to a telephone, and safety and hygiene practices.
- When assessing the patient's potential for complying with the treatment plan, consider such factors as history of psychiatric disorders, developmental status, substance abuse, comprehension, ability to read and write, and the presence of language barriers.
- OASIS isn't a substitute for a thorough assessment; it's an addition. Some agencies have integrated their assessment forms and the OASIS data tool. (See OASIS-C2 form at the CMS website: https://www.cms.gov/Medicare/Quality-Initiatives-Patient -Assessment-Instruments/HomehealthQualityInits/Downloads /OASIS-C2-AllItems-10-2016.pdf.)
- OASIS guidelines specify the questions to be asked. All must be asked, even though the patient may decline to answer some. Note the questions the patient declines to answer on your record, and report the situation to your supervisor.
- OASIS data must be electronically transmitted to CMS when complete.

Care plan

Professional standards dictated by CHAP in 1993—under the guidance of NLN—require you to develop a comprehensive individualized care plan in cooperation with the patient and caregivers.

Family counsel

In many aspects of care, the patient and family become the decision makers. This fact must be taken into account when developing your care plan; adjust your interventions, patient goals, and teaching accordingly. Reimbursement must also be considered.

Don't go astray—without documenting it, at least

Legally speaking, a care plan is the most direct evidence of your nursing judgment. If you outline a care plan and then deviate from it, a court may decide that you strayed from a reasonable standard of care. So be sure to update your care plan regularly and make sure it fits the patient's needs.

Collating care

Some agencies use the home health certification form and care plan form (required for Medicare reimbursement) as the official care plan for Medicare patients. Most home health agencies, however, require a separate care plan.

Agencies use a multidisciplinary, integrated care plan for those patients receiving more than one service such as physical or occupational therapy.

Guidelines for use

To document most effectively on your care plan, follow these suggestions:

- Keep a copy of the care plan in the patient's home for easy reference for the patient and family or caregiver.
- Make sure the plan is comprehensive by including more than the patient's physiologic problems. Also document information about the home environment, the resources needed, and the attitudes or concerns of the patient, family, and caregiver.
- Document physical changes that must be made in the patient's home in order for the patient to receive proper care. Help the family find the resources to implement them.
- Describe the primary caregiver, including whether the caregiver lives with the patient, their relationship, age and physical ability, and willingness to help the patient. The patient's well-being may depend on this person's abilities.
- Document how you made the most of the patient's strengths and resources. Strengths include support systems, good health habits and coping behaviors, a safe and healthful environment, and financial security. Resources include the practitioner, pharmacy, and medical equipment supplier.
- Document teaching provided to the patient, family, and caregiver; their understanding of that teaching; and if follow-up teaching is needed.
- Document progress or lack of progress toward established goals. If the patient is unable to make progress, discharge may be considered.
- If the patient is homebound, make sure this is documented at every visit and state the reason why. Medicare requires a patient receiving skilled home care to be homebound; however, some commercial insurers don't.
- Make sure that documentation reflects consistent adherence by all caregivers to the care plan. Have caregivers demonstrate the procedures they provide to the patient and document their skill level.
- Keep the record updated, noting changes in the patient's condition or care plan, and document that you reported these changes to the practitioner. Be sure to include the date and time of notification and the practitioner's name and response. Medicare, Medicaid, and certain other third-party payers won't reimburse for skilled services not reported to the practitioner.
- Interdisciplinary care must be documented on an ongoing basis. Collaboration on patient care problems and changes to the care plan should be described in detail in the patient's medical record.

Progress notes

The home care progress note, as with notes in the acute care setting, is a place to document the patient's condition and significant events that occur while under your care. The progress note is written in chronologic order based on each home visit. (See *Progress note.*)

With each visit, you should add a new progress note to the patient's medical record.

Work in progress

Every time you visit a patient, you must write a progress note. These notes document:
- the patient's condition, including changes, if applicable
- skilled nursing interventions you performed related to the care plan
- the patient's responses to the interventions
- events or incidents in the home that might affect the treatment plan
- patient's vital signs and pain assessment
- teaching provided to the patient and caregiver, including written instructional materials and brochures, their understanding of that teaching, and if follow-up teaching is needed
- communication with other team members since the previous visit
- any unusual events
- discharge plans
- time you arrived in the home and time you left the home.

Guidelines for use
The guidelines here will help you document accurately on progress notes:
- Chart all events in chronologic order.
- Avoid addendums.

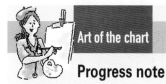

Art of the chart

Progress note

Use this sample progress note as a guide when documenting in home care settings.

Date	Problem no.	Problem title—subjective, objective, assessment, plan
2/6/2017	#2	A: ① foot stasis ulcer showing no improvement in size or amount of drainage since 2/1/2017 P: Dr. T. Miller notified. Wound culture ordered and collected; sent specimen to lab ———— M. A. Ford, RN

- Provide a heading for each entry because many members of the health care team use the progress notes.
- Use flow sheets and checklists to record vital signs, intake and output measurements, and nutritional data per agency policy. Encourage the patient or caregiver to fill out these forms when appropriate to promote participation in care and increase the patient's feeling of control.
- When possible, take time to complete your documentation in the home while the information is fresh in your mind. This decreases the chance that information is forgotten or omitted from the patient's medical record.
- Encourage the patient to be involved with the care and documentation by making statements like, "Here's what I've written about how your wound is healing. Is there anything else you want me to put in the notes?"
- If the patient has a medical emergency while you're there, contact emergency medical services and stay until the paramedics take over. Call the practitioner for transport orders. Notify your supervisor, who'll arrange coverage for your other patients, if necessary. Document all assessments, interventions performed, and patient response to interventions, until you're relieved. Note the date and time of transfer and the name of the caregiver who assumes responsibility.

Patient teaching

Correct documentation will help justify to your agency and to third-party payers your visits to provide teaching to the patient or caregiver. Identify the patient's and family's needs, resources, and support systems to help outline the basic teaching plan.

Keeping continuity

Remember that teaching is usually an ongoing process requiring more than one visit. Until the patient becomes independent, your documentation will help other nurses continue or reinforce the teaching and identify additional areas of teaching needed. (See *Certification of instruction*, page 249.)

Keep a list of teaching and reference materials you have supplied to the patient or caregiver. Also document modifications made to accommodate the patient's or caregiver's literacy skills and native language.

Being there

If the patient isn't physically or mentally able to perform skills and a caregiver is not available, report

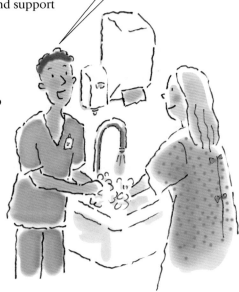

Be there for a patient until the patient is able to perform a procedure adequately without assistance.

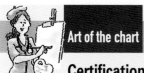

Art of the chart

Certification of instruction

The model patient-teaching form below shows what was taught to a home-care patient with an intravenous (I.V.) catheter. This type of form will help you document your teaching sessions clearly and completely.

CONTENT (check all that apply; fill in blanks as indicated)

1. ☐ Reason for therapy

2. Drug/Solution
   ☐ Dose
   ☐ Schedule
   ☐ Label accuracy
   ☐ Storage
   ☐ Container integrity

3. Aseptic technique
   ☐ Hand washing
   ☐ Prepping caps/connections
   ☐ Tubing/cap/needs
   ☐ Needless adaptor changes

4. Access device maintenance
   Type/Name: _____
   ☒ Device/Site Inspection
   ☐ Site care/Dsg. changes
   ☐ Catheter clamping
   ☒ Maintaining patency
      ☒ Saline flushing
      ☐ Heparin locking
      ☐ Fdg. Tube /declogging
      ☐ Self insertion of device

5. Drug preparation
   ☒ Premixed containers
   ☐ Compounding
   ☐ Client additives
   ☐ Piggyback lipids

6. Method of administration
   ☐ Gravity
   ☒ Pump (name): _CADD pump_
   ☐ Continuous   ☒ Intermittent
   ☐ Cycle/Taper:

7. Administration technique
   ☒ Pump rate/calibration
   ☐ Priming tubing   ☐ Filter
   ☐ Filling syringe
   ☐ Loading pump
   ☒ Access device hookup/disconnect

8. Potential complications/Adverse effects
   ☐ Patient drug information sheet reviewed
   ☒ Pump alarms/troubleshooting
   ☒ Phlebitis/infiltration
   ☐ Clotting/dislodgment
   ☒ Infection   ☐ Air embolus
   ☐ Breakage/cracking
   ☐ Electrolyte imbalance
   ☐ Fluid balance
   ☐ Glucose intolerance
   ☐ Aspiration
   ☐ N / V / D / Cramping
   ☐ Other: _____

9. Self-monitoring:
   ☐ Weight   ☒ Temperature   ☐ P   ☐ PB
   ☐ Urine S & A   ☐ Fingersticks
   ☐ Other: _____

10 Supply handling/disposal
   ☒ Disposal of sharps/supplies   ☐ Opioids
   ☐ Cleaning pump
   ☒ Changing batteries
   ☐ Blood/fluid precautions
   ☐ Chemo/spill precautions

11 Information given to client re:
   ☐ Pharmacy counseling
   ☐ Advance directives
   ☐ Inventory checks
   ☐ Deliveries
   ☒ 24-hour on-call staff
   ☒ Reimbursement
   ☐ Service complaints

12 Safety/Disaster plan
   ☐ Back up pump batteries
   ☒ Emergency room use
   ☐ Electrical
   ☒ Disaster
   ☐ Other:

13 Written instructions
   ☒ Yes   ☐ No   If, no why? _____
   _____
   _____
   _____
   _____

This document helps ensure continuity of patient teaching.

☐ Client or caregiver demonstrates or verbalizes competency to perform home infusion therapy.

COMMENTS: _Wife incorrectly changed pump battery. Procedure reviewed. Wife then demonstrated correct procedure. Wife also concerned about frequency of dressing changes. Access site nonreddened and not edematous. Protocol reviewed. Pt states he is satisfied with waiting until scheduled dressing change tomorrow._

The form provides room to comment and document individual instructions.

Theory/Skill reviewed/Return demonstration completed:

Chris Banner, RN   2/14/2017
Signature of RN Educator   **Date**

CERTIFICATION OF INSTRUCTION

I agree that I have been instructed as described above and understand that the above functions will be performed in the home by myself and caregiver, out-side a hospital or medically supervised environment.

Robert Burns   2/14/2017
Client/Caregiver signature   **Date**

In this part of the form, the patient acknowledges responsibility for self-care activities.

this in your documentation. The patient most likely isn't an appropriate candidate for home care. Never leave a patient alone to perform a procedure until the patient can express understanding of it and perform it competently.

Setting the terms (on the packages)

Be careful to call equipment by the same names used on the packages and in teaching literature. Consider providing a glossary of terms and labeling machines to match your instructions. Make sure that the patient can identify devices when speaking on the telephone. Document all teaching materials given to the patient, and keep copies of teaching materials in your records. You may want to videotape your instructions in the home if more than one caregiver will be providing care.

Signing off

Most agencies require patients to sign a teaching documentation record indicating that they accept responsibility for learning self-care activities. This documentation is a critical piece of the home care chart.

Nursing and discharge summaries

As a home health nurse, you must submit a regular patient progress report to the attending practitioner and to the reimburser to confirm the need for continuing services. You must also complete a summary of the patient's progress and a discharge summary.

Summing it all up

When writing a summary of the patient's progress, include:
- current problems, treatments, interventions, and instructions
- home care provided by other health care professionals, such as a physical therapist or speech pathologist
- the reason for a change in services
- patient outcomes and responses—physical and emotional—to the services provided
- discharge plan.

Guidelines for use

You'll prepare a discharge summary for the practitioner's approval to discharge a patient, to notify third-party payers that services have been terminated, and to officially close the case. The discharge summary also serves as a brief history for quick review if the patient is readmitted at a later date.

When writing these summaries, record:

- time frame covered
- services provided and the names and titles of assigned staff
- clinical and psychosocial conditions of the patient at discharge
- recommendations for further care
- caregiver involvement in care
- interruptions in home care such as readmissions to the hospital
- referrals to community agencies
- OASIS discharge information
- patient's response to and comprehension of patient-teaching efforts
- outcomes attained.

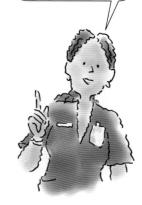

In your summary of the patient's progress, document the patient's physical and emotional responses to care.

Medicare-mandated forms

CMS, the federal watchdog agency that oversees Medicare and Medicaid programs, requires home health agencies that receive Medicare funding to standardize their record keeping and documentation methods. Home health agencies must maintain the following forms for each qualified Medicare recipient:

- OASIS
- home health certification and plan of care (See *Home Health Certification and Plan of Care form*, page 252.)
- medical update and patient information (See *Medical Update and Patient Information form*, page 253.)
- notice of nondiscrimination
- privacy notice.

Practitioner calls

In addition, home care nurses must document the practitioner's telephone orders. The Joint Commission requires that you write the practitioner's order verbatim, note the date and time, and write "V.T.O." (verified telephone order) on the order form, which means that you read back the order and received confirmation that it's correct. If this documentation is not entered via an electronic health system for practitioner's orders, complete an order using the agency approved paperwork. (See *Practitioner's telephone orders*, page 254.)

Fill out and sign, please . . .

Medicare, via the fiscal intermediary, won't provide reimbursement unless the required forms are properly completed, signed, and submitted. Forms are usually completed by the nurse assigned to the patient, although some agencies have an admission team and a care team.

(Text continues on page 254.)

Art of the chart

Home Health Certification and Plan of Care form

The form below is the official form for authorizing Medicare coverage for home care (also known as form 485). It includes space for assessing functional abilities and documenting care plan information.

HOME HEALTH CERTIFICATION AND PLAN OF CARE

4. Medical Record No. 78-9101	5. Provider No. 11-1213

2. Start Of Care Date 2/08/2017

3. Certification Period From: 2/08/2017 To: 4/08/2017

1. Patient's HI Claim No. 111-111

7. Provider's Name, Address and Telephone Number
Home Health Agency
301 Main St.
Wichita, Kansas 67202

6. Patient's Name and Address
Mary Long
2218 Central Ave.
Wichita, Kansas 67202

9. Sex M ☐ F ☒

10. Medications: Dose/Frequency/Route (N)ew (C)hanged
digoxin 0.125 mg P.O. daily; Lasix 20 mg P.O. daily; warfarin 5mg P.O. daily; Capoten 12.5 mg b.i.d.; Proventil inh 2 puffs q.i.d. p.r.n.; MVI one P.O. daily; FeSO₄ 325 mg daily; Ex St Tylenol 500 mg q4h p.r.n.; albuterol 0.5cc with 3 ml ns via nebulizer b.i.d.; 325 mg aspirin P.O. daily:

> To maintain Medicare coverage, complete this form and submit it for approval every 60 days.

8. Date of Birth 06/04/29

11. ICD-9-CM Principal Diagnosis atrial fibrillation 4273l
Date 01/1/2017

12. ICD-9-CM Surgical Procedure gastrostomy tube insertion 0000
Date 10/3/2016

13. ICD-9-CM Other Pertinent Diagnoses
4280 heart failure
496 chr airway obstruct
Date 10/1/2016   11/29/2016

15. Safety Measures: prevent falls; emergency, fire response, and disaster plan

14. DME and Supplies gastrostomy tube supplies, cane

17. Allergies: NKA

16. Nutritional Req. magnacal 80 ml per hr

18.B. Activities Permitted
1 ☐ Complete Bedrest
2 ☐ Bedrest BRP
3 ☐ Up As Tolerated
4 ☐ Transfer Bed/Chair
5 ☐ Exercises Prescribed
6 ☐ Partial Weight Bearing
7 ☐ Independent At Home
8 ☐ Crutches
9 ☑ Cane
A ☐ Wheelchair
B ☐ Walker
C ☐ No Restrictions
D ☐ Other (Specify)

18.A. Functional Limitations
1 ☐ Amputation
2 ☐ Bowel/Bladder (Incontinence)
3 ☐ Contracture
4 ☐ Hearing
5 ☐ Paralysis
6 ☑ Endurance
7 ☐ Ambulation
8 ☐ Speech
9 ☐ Legally Blind
A ☐ Dyspnea With Minimal Exertion
B ☐ Other (Specify)

19. Mental Status:
1 ☑ Oriented
2 ☐ Comatose
3 ☐ Forgetful
4 ☐ Depressed
5 ☐ Disoriented
6 ☐ Lethargic
7 ☐ Agitated
8 ☐ Other

20. Prognosis:
1 ☐ Poor
2 ☐ Guarded
3 ☐ Fair
4 ☑ Good
5 ☐ Excellent

21. Orders for Discipline and Treatments (Specify Amount/Frequency/Duration)
RN: assess heart failure, effects of digoxin, monitor complaints of arthritis pain control; monitor gastrostomy tube site, help with gastrostomy feedings and tube care 5-7x/wk for 9 weeks. Draw blood as ordered by MD. AID 2-3wk for 9 weeks; assist with personal care and ADLs.

> Note that a patient is required to be homebound to receive Medicare reimbursement.

22. Goals/Rehabilitation Potential/Discharge Plans
Pt needs teaching reinforcement and emotional support for colostomy. Rehab potential is good. Discharge to independent ADLs.

23. Nurse's Signature and Date of Verbal SOC Where Applicable: N. Smith, RN 2/08/2017

25. Date HHA Received Signed POT 2/08/2017

26. I certify/recertify that this patient is confined to his/her home and needs intermittent skilled nursing care, physical therapy and/or speech therapy or continues to need occupational therapy. The patient is under my care, and I have authorized the services on this plan of care and will periodically review the plan.

24. Physician's Name and Address M. Raser, MD 555 S. Main St. Wichita, Kansas 67202

28. Anyone who misrepresents, falsifies, or conceals essential information required for payment of Federal funds may be subject to fine, imprisonment, or civil penalty under applicable Federal laws.

27. Attending Physician's Signature and Date Signed
M. Raser, MD

PROVIDER

Form HCFA-485 (C-4) (02-94) (Print Aligned)

Art of the chart

Medical Update and Patient Information form

To continue providing reimbursable skilled nursing care to a patient at home, Medicare requires you to complete the Medical Update and Patient Information form (also known as form 486).

Form Approved
OMB No. 0938-0357

MEDICAL UPDATE AND PATIENT INFORMATION

Department of Health and Human Services
Health Care Financing Administration

| | | | 4. Medical Record No. 00-0000 | 5. Provider No. 98-7654 |

1. Patient's HI Claim No. 48-7850
2. SOC Date 2/5/2017
3. Certification Period From: 2/5/2017 To: 3/5/2017
7. Provider's Name Home Health Agency

6. Patient's Name and Address James Dole, Main Street, Newark, NJ 07105

8. Medicare Covered: ☑Y ☐N
9. Date Physician Last Saw Patient: 2/10/2017
10. Date Last Contacted Physician: 2/20/2017

11. Is the Patient Receiving Care in an 1861 (J)(1) Skilled Nursing Facility or Equivalent? ☐Y ☑N ☐ Do Not Know

12. ☐ Certification ☐ Recertification ☐ Modified

14. Type of Facility: A

13. Dates of Last Inpatient Stay: Admission 12/01/2016   Discharge 12/05/2016

15. Updated information: New Orders/Treatments/Clinical Facts/Summary from Each Discipline

Discipline	Visits (this bill)	Frequency and duration	Treatment codes	Total visits projected this cert.
			A01 A06	07
SN	00	2M0203	F04	27
ADL	00	3WK09		

SN A&O x 3. Skin warm, dry, pale, slight dyspnea noted with activity. Trace bilat. pedal edema, lungs clear. No complaints. Improved & increased feeling of well-being demonstrated. Peg tube patent and functioning well. Correctly demonstrates checking for residual, peg tube site care.
AID pt seen 3x/wk. Increased difficulty ambulating. Expressed feelings of despair and hopelessness associated with physical condition.

16. Functional Limitations (Expand From 485 and Level of ADL) Reason Homebound/Prior Functional Status
Interaction between pt and daughter who wants pt to strive to live. Pt increasingly fearful of institutional care. Pt agrees to gastrostomy support group. CCSW to facilitate. Needs more encouragement to perform ADLs. Daughter more involved with care.   ☐Y ☐N

17. Supplementary Plan of Care on File from Physician Other than Referring Physician:
(If Yes, Please Specify Giving Goals/Rehab. Potential/Discharge Plan)

18. Unusual Home/Social Environment   N/A

19. Indicate Any Time When the Home Health Agency Made a Visit and Patient was Not Home and Reason Why if Ascertainable

20. Specify Any Known Medical and/or Non-Medical Reasons the Patient Regularly Leaves Home and Frequency of Occurrence

Date (Mo., Day, Yr.) 3/5/2017

21. Nurse or Therapist Completing or Reviewing Form   M. Hoffner, RN

PROVIDER

Form HCFA-486 (C3) (02-94) (Print Aligned)

To maintain Medicare approval, this form must be completed after the first 60 days of care and submitted with the Home Health Certification and Plan of Care form.

Note that this form is multidisciplinary. It includes charting by a skilled nurse, physical and occupational therapists, an SLP, and an MSW.

Don't leave any blank spaces.

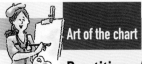

Art of the chart

Practitioner's telephone orders

Home health nurses rely heavily on the use of telephone orders. The agency must follow guidelines established by the Centers for Medicare & Medicaid Services and The Joint Commission for taking and documenting these orders. Below is an example of a form used by one agency to fulfill documentation requirements.

Facility name		Address		Admission no.
Suburban Home Health Agency		123 Main Street		
Last name	**First name**	**Attending practitioner**		**Admission no.**
Smith	Kevin	Dr. Michael Baker		147-111-471

Date ordered	Date discontinued	ORDERS
2/10/2017	2/13/2017	Tylenol 650 mg P.O. q 6h

> The order must be signed by the practitioner within 48 hours.

Signature of nurse receiving order	Time	Signature of practitioner	Date
V.T.O/Mary Reo, RN	1820		

Future developments

Several major trends are emerging as the home health care industry continues to evolve:

- More private insurers require preauthorization for home health care services, which increases the paperwork burden for nurses.
- Fewer visits per episode of care are allowed. More focused reimbursement will dramatically alter the amount of home care patients will receive.
- The depth and breadth of federal regulations have placed increasing demands on care providers, and agencies need to computerize record keeping.
- Telehealth technology is being used by home health agencies to monitor patients in their homes via telephone communication. Nurses are able to help patients with chronic conditions using twice-per-week "visits" to identify the need for or help avoid

hospitalization. Telehealth offers an ideal way to care for patients at home.
- Family caregivers will be assessed for ability, willingness, and availability to participate in the patient's care. This will help the nurse develop a more accurate plan of care.

One predicted outcome: More reliance on outcomes

Increased reliance on disease-specific management programs will eventually lead to the use of care pathways that incorporate patient outcomes in home health care. Both CMS and The Joint Commission are focused on outcomes. State departments of health services surveyors also have access to data. In addition, an agency's data are compared with data from similar agencies.

Computers at work

Home health care nurses are commonly using laptop computers or handheld devices equipped with software designed to speed clinical documentation. Many of these programs are designed to help nurses develop a care plan, formulate goals, monitor patient progress, update medications, and generate visit notes.

This technology expedites the exchange of data between care providers and third-party payers and is often the required method of communication.

Keeping it confidential

Technology changes every day, and this raises concerns about confidentiality. For example, e-mails, texts, and faxes can easily end up being viewed by the wrong individual. When using any electronic method to transmit information about a patient, consider blacking out or omitting identifying data. Arrange for the recipient of a fax to wait at the other end for the fax to print.

Confidentiality when transmitting OASIS data on patients who aren't Medicare recipients continues to be a source of concern. Legislators and lawmakers will ultimately reconcile the parameters of government access to non-Medicare patients' clinical data.

In many cases, a home health agency will supply its nurses with laptop computers to streamline documentation and provide security for the information entered. Laptop computers shouldn't be used by anyone other than agency personnel. You may be tempted to allow a computer-savvy spouse, friend, or child to add programs or manipulate data with all good intentions, but this is no more appropriate than it would be to let them read a patient's record. Finally, access to computer files should be protected by a strong password to prevent unauthorized individuals from entering files.

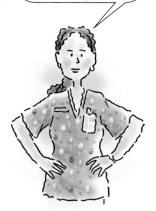

Laptop computers help streamline documentation of home health care.

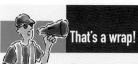
That's a wrap!

Home health care documentation review

The basics
You must become familiar with many forms unique to home care. For each visit, documentation includes:
• assessment
• interventions
• patient's treatment and response to treatment
• teaching and complications.

Legal risks and responsibilities
• Risks of poor documentation or inadequate or incomplete documentation may result in a lawsuit or refusal by third-party payers to cover services.

Documentation guidelines
• Careful screening will determine what services the patient needs.
• Document activities completed during your nursing visits, including assessments, interventions, patient's response, and complications.
• Include evidence that the home environment is safe.
• Document emergency and resource numbers given to the patient or caregiver.
• Document teaching provided and the patient's or caregiver's ability to perform procedures, troubleshoot equipment, and recognize potential complications and respond appropriately.

Home health care forms
• *Agency assessment and Outcome and Assessment Information Set (OASIS) forms* provide information on a thorough patient assessment needed to plan appropriate care.
• A *care plan* is required by professional standards and is the most direct evidence of your nursing judgment.
• *Progress notes* are written in chronologic order and are the place to document the patient's condition and significant events that occur.
• *Patient teaching* is an ongoing process until the patient becomes independent. Correct documentation will help justify your visits.
• *Nursing and discharge summaries* are summaries of the patient's progress. A discharge summary must be submitted to the practitioner and the reimburser.
• *Medicare-mandated forms* include an OASIS form, a Home Health Care Certification form, a care plan, and a Medical Update and Patient Information form.

Trends
• Major documentation trends continue to evolve, including preauthorization for services, fewer visits allowed per episode, increasing federal regulations, and use of telehealth technology.
• Increased reliance on disease-specific management programs can lead to care pathways and outcomes incorporation.
• Laptop computers and handheld devices speed documentation and increase concerns about confidentiality.

Suggested references

Carpenito, L.J. *Nursing Care Plans: Transitional Patient & Family Centered Care*, 7th ed. Philadelphia, PA: Lippincott Williams & Wilkins, 2017.

Centers for Medicare & Medicaid Services. "Home Health Certification and Plan of Care," n.d. Available: https://www.cdc.gov/wtc/pdfs/CMS-485.pdf.

Centers for Medicare & Medicaid Services. "Medical Update and Patient Information," n.d. Available: http://www.staffhospital.com/sites/default/files/fieldStaff Forms/CMS%20487.pdf.

Centers for Medicare & Medicaid Services. "OASIS-C2 All Timepoints Item Set," 2017. Available: https://www.cms.gov/Medicare/Quality-Initiatives-Patient -Assessment-Instruments/HomeHealthQualityInits/Downloads/OASIS-C2 -AllItems-10-2016.pdf.

Centers for Medicare & Medicaid Services. "Outcome and Assessment Information Set: Oasis-C2 Guidance Manual" 2018. Available: https://www.cms.gov /Medicare/Quality-Initiatives-Patient-Assessment-Instruments /HomeHealthQualityInits/Downloads/OASIS-C2-Guidance-Manual -Effective_1_1_18.pdf.

Community Health Accreditation Partner. "2018 CHAP Standards of Excellence v.1 for Home Health Providers," 2017. Available: http://www.chapinc.org /chap-standards-of-excellence/2018-chap-standards-of-excellence.aspx.

Vossel, H. (Ed). *2017 Joint Commission & CMS Crosswalk: Comparing Hospital Standards and CoPs*. Oak Brook, IL: Joint Commission Resources, 2017.

Chapter 11

Long-term care documentation

Just the facts

In this chapter, you'll learn:

♦ documentation regulation and requirements for long-term care settings

♦ guidelines for correct documentation in long-term care.

A look at documenting in long-term care

A long-term care facility provides continuing care for chronically ill or disabled patients. The purpose of care is to promote the highest level of functioning possible for the patient. Long-term care is an increasingly important form of health care delivery, especially because the elderly segment of the population continues to grow. (See *Elder power*, page 259.)

Maintaining accurate, complete documentation in long-term care is vital. Consider the following points:

• Long-term care facilities are highly regulated by state and federal agencies and therefore must adhere to high standards of documentation.

• Information that you document may be used to defend you and your facility in a lawsuit.

• Documentation is considered evidence of standardized, high-quality nursing care.

• Good record keeping ensures certification, licensure, reimbursement, and accreditation.

Documentation distinctions

Two key differences exist between documenting in long-term care settings and documenting in other settings:

1. Patients stay at long-term care facilities for weeks, months, or even years, so documentation isn't done as often, which provides more time to care for the patient or help the patient relearn basic skills.

2. Some of the government forms used in long-term facilities are long and involved. So, even though documentation isn't emphasized, it can still be extensive.

Elder power

According to the 2010 U.S. Census, 40.3 million people—13% of the total population—were age 65 years or older in 2010, with an estimate of 15.2% of the population being older than age 65 years in 2016. Among the older population, 21.7 million people were ages 65 to 74 years, 13.1 million people were ages 75 to 84 years, and 5.4 million people were 85 years or older. The older population will continue to increase; the older-than-85 years population is estimated to reach 8.9 million by 2030.

Chances are, you're caring for many elderly patients right now. Studies show that people age 65 years and older require health care services more often than any other age-group. Most older people have at least one chronic condition and many have coexisting conditions. That's why we need to increase focus on the needs of elderly patients, not only in long-term care but in all health care settings.

There's strength in numbers!

Categories of care

Long-term care facilities usually offer two levels of care: skilled and intermediate. The level of care administered to your patient should be your primary consideration when documenting.

Care may be complex . . .

In a skilled care facility, patient care involves specialized nursing skills, such as intravenous (I.V.) therapy, parenteral nutrition, respiratory care, and mechanical ventilation.

. . . or not so complex

An intermediate care facility deals with patients who have chronic illnesses and need less complex care. For example, they may simply need assistance with activities of daily living (ADLs), such as bathing and dressing.

Patients at both levels may need short- or long-term care and may move from one level to another according to their progress or decline. Living arrangements, geography, family and community support networks, and other factors determine the patient's length of stay.

Regulatory agencies

Documentation in long-term care facilities is regulated by federal and state agencies. Documentation is influenced by:
- federal programs, such as Medicare and Medicaid
- government agencies such as the Centers for Medicare & Medicaid Services (CMS)

- laws such as the Omnibus Budget Reconciliation Act (OBRA) of 1987
- state regulations for each facility
- accrediting agencies, such as The Joint Commission and the Commission on Accreditation of Rehabilitation Facilities (CARF).

Most elderly patients entering long-term care facilities pay for the services privately. When their funds become exhausted, they apply to Medicaid for coverage. If the patient requires services and is unable to pay initially, an application can be submitted to receive Medicaid.

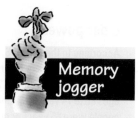

Memory jogger

To remember the conditions that affect length of stay, think of the word **FOCUS**:

Functional skills (and disabilities)

Other diseases

Chronicity

Urgency of needs

Support systems.

Medicare

Few of the services provided in long-term care facilities are eligible for Medicare reimbursement. However, Medicare does provide reimbursement for patients requiring skilled care, such as chemotherapy, tube feeding, and certain types of wound care. For these patients, Medicare requires certain minimum daily documentation to verify that a service was needed. If the patient's status changes, you must supply a revised care plan within 7 days.

Making reimbursement a reality

Be sure to document changes in status when a patient who isn't improving or expected to improve according to the care plan is ineligible for coverage. You must also document the need for new or continuing skilled services you provide. Medicare also requires documentation of your evaluations for expected outcomes.

According to Medicare guidelines, documentation must clearly show that a patient needed care by a professional or technical staff member. To verify the need for skilled rehabilitative care, you must describe a reasonable expectation of improvement or services needed to establish a maintenance program. The amount, duration, and frequency of services must be reasonable and necessary.

> Medicare does cover some skilled services in long-term care, but daily documentation is required.

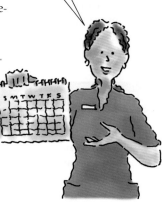

Medicaid

Most patients who receive skilled care in long-term care facilities either pay for it themselves or are on Medicaid. To ensure Medicaid reimbursement for these patients, document patient care once per day.

Reimbursement for intermediate care

To secure payment for patients receiving intermediate care, medications and treatments are documented daily. Document other types of care weekly, unless the patient's status changes and requiring a change in services. In this case, document the change and the patient's status more frequently. Also, perform a monthly reevaluation for these patients and an evaluation of expected outcomes for all Medicaid patients.

CMS and Resident Assessment Instrument

A branch of the U.S. Department of Health and Human Services, CMS regulates compliance with federal Medicare and Medicaid standards. CMS regulations are usually enforced at the state level.

To comply with CMS regulations, staff members at a long-term care facility must utilize the Resident Assessment Instrument (RAI) with completion for any resident residing more than 14 days in a facility. The purpose of the RAI is to assist the long-term care facility staff in collecting information regarding a resident's strengths and needs, evaluating that information, and formulating an individualized patient care plan. The components of the RAI include a lengthy form called the Minimum Data Set (MDS) for Resident Assessment and Care Screening; the care area assessment (CAA) process, which is an interpretation of the information on the MDS and assists with creating a care plan; and utilization guidelines, which provides information regarding how and when to use the RAI.

OBRA

In 1987, Congress enacted OBRA (Omnibus Budget Reconciliation Act), which imposed dozens of new requirements on long-term care facilities and home health agencies to protect the rights of patients receiving long-term care. OBRA requires that a comprehensive assessment be performed within 7 days of a patient's admission to a long-term care facility and then be documented on the MDS form. The assessment and care screening process must be reviewed every 3 months and repeated annually—more often if the patient's condition changes.

In addition, a comprehensive nursing assessment and a formulated care plan must be completed. The comprehensive care plan must be completed within 7 days of the completion of the MDS. This date may vary depending on whether it's a Medicare Prospective Payment System (PPS) or an intermediate assessment.

The Joint Commission

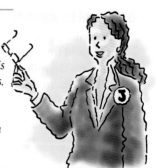

The Joint Commission accredits long-term care facilities using standards developed in conjunction with health care experts. Standard performance is documented in assessments, progress notes, care plans, and discharge plans. The ORYX initiative, begun in 1997, is another part of the accreditation process. It focuses on outcomes and other performance measurement data. The purpose of the initiative is to support quality improvements, not just in long-term care but in all health care organizations.

Forms used in long-term care

Many forms are used in acute care and home health care settings as well as in long-term care; others are used only in long-term care. Forms discussed in this chapter include:
- Preadmission Screening and Annual Resident Review (PASARR)
- MDS
- initial nursing assessment form
- nursing summaries
- ADL checklists or flow sheets
- care plans
- discharge and transfer forms.

In addition, many long-term care facilities have their own strict and comprehensive protocols. Typical protocols are those for bowel and bladder monitoring, physical and chemical restraints, safety, and infection control. Documentation requirements when using these protocols vary, so check your facility's policies.

MDS

Mandated by OBRA, the MDS is a federal regulatory form that must be filled out for every patient admitted to a long-term care facility. (See Minimum Data Set form at the CMS website: https://www.cms .gov/Medicare/Quality-Initiatives-Patient-Assessment-Instruments /NursingHomeQualityInits/Downloads/Archive-Draft-of-the-MDS -30-Nursing-Home-Comprehensive-NC-Version-1140.pdf.)

The MDS form proves compliance with quality improvement and reimbursement requirements, standardizes information, and helps health care team members and agencies communicate. Practitioners, nurses, social workers, and other staff members complete and sign different sections of the form. There are different forms available based on when they are being completed. Forms can be found at the CMS website: https://www.cms.gov/Medicare/Quality-Initiatives-Patient-Assessment -Instruments/NursingHomeQualityInits/MDS30RAIManual.html.

The requirements for completion of the MDS vary with the type of admission and can be complex. Most assessments are completed at these times:

- admission assessment—required by day 14
- annual assessment
- significant change in status assessment
- quarterly review assessment—performed every 3 months.

CAA

When an MDS form is completed, coded, computed, and processed, CAAs are triggered specific to the patient's primary problems, needs or strengths. Interpretation of these triggers is the basis of the CAA process which assists with providing information to develop an individualized care plan for the patient. There are 20 care areas that have been established and commonly identified by MDS findings. Further development of a care plan based on the CAA should follow evidence-based practice and specific facility guidelines. (See *Care area assessments*.)

Care area assessments

After completion and processing of a Minimum Data Set (MDS), care area assessments (CAAs) may be triggered that should be addressed to confirm a patient's problem or need, with the subsequent development of a care plan specifically developed for the patient. Twenty established CAAs include:

- delirium
- cognitive loss/dementia
- visual function
- communication
- activities of daily living (ADLs) functional/rehabilitation potential
- urinary incontinence/indwelling catheter
- psychosocial well-being
- mood state
- behavioral symptoms
- activities
- falls
- nutritional status
- feeding tubes
- dehydration/fluid management
- dental care
- pressure ulcer
- psychotropic medication use
- physical restraints
- pain
- return to community referral

Source: Centers for Medicare & Medicaid Services. "Long-Term Care Facility Resident Assessment Instrument 3.0 User's Manual. Version 1.15," 2017. Available: https://downloads.cms.gov/files/MDS-30-RAI-Manual-v115-October-2017.pdf.

PASARR

All patients who apply for admission to a long-term care facility must be evaluated for serious mental illness (SMI) and/or an intellectual disability (ID), called a Level I PASARR screening. If it is determined that the patient may have an SMI or ID, then a more in-depth evaluation is performed, called a Level II PASARR screening. These screenings help determine the patient's best placement for long-term care. (See *Preadmission Screening and Annual Resident Review Level I Screening form*, pages 265 to 268.)

Initial nursing assessment

This required form is similar to the initial assessment form used in other settings. When documenting your initial assessment in a long-term care setting, place special emphasis on the patient's:
- activity level
- hearing and vision
- bowel and bladder control
- nutrition and hydration status
- ability to communicate
- safety
- need for adaptive devices to assist dexterity and mobility
- family relationships
- transition from home or hospital to the long-term care facility.

Nursing summaries

Care and status updates must be completed regularly in long-term care facilities. Usually, you must complete a standard nursing care summary at least once every 2 to 4 weeks for patients with specific problems, such as pressure injuries, who are receiving skilled care. A summary addressing the specific problems must be done weekly. For patients receiving intermediate care, a standard nursing care summary is usually required every 4 weeks.

Summing it up

The nursing summary describes:
- the patient's ability to perform ADLs
- nutrition and hydration
- safety measures, such as bed rails, restraints, or adaptive devices
- medications and other treatments
- problems the patient has adjusting to the long-term care facility.
  In addition, you must complete a nursing assessment summary at least monthly to comply with Medicare and Medicaid standards.

(Text continues on page 268.)

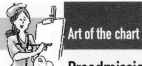

Art of the chart

Preadmission Screening and Annual Resident Review Level I Screening form

Before a patient covered by Medicare or Medicaid enters a long-term care facility, an evaluation of mental status must be completed, using the Preadmission Screening and Annual Resident Review (PASARR) Level I Screening form shown here. *Note: PASARR forms may vary by state.*

SECTION A. IDENTIFYING INFORMATION FOR APPLICANT/RESIDENT

Last name	First name	MI
Perrone	Joseph	R

Sex M = Male F = Female	Date of birth	Social security number	Medicaid Recipient?	Y = Yes N = No P = Pending
M	08/10/33	012345678	N	

SECTION B: REASON FOR SCREENING

Enter code: **1**

Preadmission Screening Codes
1-Nursing Facility Applicant
2-PASSPORT Waiver Applicant

Annual RESIDENT REVIEW CODES
3-Expired Time Limit for Convalescent Stay
4-Expired Time for Emergency Admission

5-Expired Time Limit for Respite Admission
6-Significant Change in Condition
7-No Previous PASARR Records

8-ODMH Use Only
9-Other

SECTION C: DEMENTIA QUESTIONS

Yes ☐ No ☑ (1) Does the individual have a documented PRIMARY diagnosis of dementia, Alzheimer's disease, or some other organic mental disorder as defined in *DSM-IV-TR*? If YES, the individual does not have indications of serious MI, go to Section E. If NO, go to the next question.

Yes ☐ No ☑ (2) Does the individual have a SECONDARY diagnosis of dementia, Alzheimer's disease, or some other organic mental disorder as defined in *DSM-IV-TR*? If YES, go to the next question. If NO, go to Section D.

Yes ☐ No ☑ (3) Does the individual have a PRIMARY diagnosis of one of the mental disorders listen in Question D (1) below? If YES, go to Section D. If NO, and the individual does not have indications of serious MI, go to Section E.

SECTION D: INDICATIONS OF SERIOUS MENTAL ILLNESS

Yes ☐ No ☐ (1) Does the individual have a diagnosis of any of the mental disorders listed below? Check all that apply.

a. ☐ Schizophrenic Disorder
b. ☐ Mood Disorder
c. ☐ Delusional (Paranoid) Disorder
d. ☐ Panic or Other Severe Anxiety Disorder

e. ☐ Somatoform Disorder
f. ☐ Personality Disorder
g. ☐ Other Psychotic Disorder
h. ☐ Another Mental Disorder Other Than MR That May Lead to a Chronic Disability
Describe: _____

> If the patient is diagnosed as having a serious mental disorder, document the diagnosis here.

Yes ☐ No ☐

OR

Yes ☐ No ☐ (b) Had a disruption to his/her usual living arrangement (e.g., arrest, eviction, inter- or intra-facility transfer, locked seclusion)? If YES, answer YES to Question D(2).

(continued)

Preadmission Screening and Annual Resident Review Level I Screening form *(continued)*

SECTION D: INDICATIONS OF SERIOUS MENTAL ILLNESS *(continued)*

Yes ☐ No ☐ (3) Within the past 6 months, DUE TO THE MENTAL DISORDER, has the individual experienced one or more of the following functional limitations on a continuing or intermittent basis? Check all that apply.

a. ☐	Maintaining Personal Hygiene	e. ☐	Preparing or Obtaining Own Meals	i. ☐	Using Available Transportation
b. ☐	Dressing Self	f. ☐	Maintaining Prescribed Medication Regimen	j. ☐	Managing Available Funds
c. ☐	Walking or Getting Around	g. ☐	Performing Household Chores	k. ☐	Securing Necessary Support Services
d. ☐	Maintaining Adequate Diet	h. ☐	Going Shopping	l. ☐	Verbalizing Needs

Yes ☐ No ☐ (4) Within the past 2 years, has the individual received SSI or SSDI due to a mental impairment?

Yes ☐ No ☐ (5) Does the individual have indications of serious mental illness?
The individual has indications of serious mental illness if the individual received:
- *Yes to AT LEAST 2 of Questions D(1), D(2), or D(3); OR*
- *Yes to Question D(4).*

> Fill out this section if the patient has mental retardation or a related condition.

SECTION E: INDICATIONS OF MR OR RELATED CONDITION

Yes ☐ No ☑ (1) Does the individual have a diagnosis of mental retardation (mild, moderate, severe, or profound as described in the *American Association of Mental Retardation's Manual on Classification in Mental Retardation*, 1989)?

Yes ☐ No ☑ (2) Does the individual have a severe, chronic disability that is attributable to a condition other than mental illness but is closely related to MR because this condition results in impairment of general intellectual functioning or adaptive behavior similar to that of a person with MR and requires treatment or services similar to those required for persons with MR? If YES, specify: _____
If NO, go to question E(6).

Yes ☐ No ☐ (3) Did the disability manifest symptoms before the individual's 22nd birthday?

Yes ☐ No ☐ (4) Is the disability likely to continue indefinitely?

Yes ☐ No ☐

Yes ☐ No ☑ (6) Does the person currently receive services from the County Board of MR/DD?

Yes ☐ No ☑ (7) Does the person have indications of MR or a related condition?

The individual has indications of MR or a related condition if the individual received:
- *Yes to Question E(1); OR*
- *Yes to all of the following in this Section; Questions 2, 3, 4 AND 5; OR*
- *Yes to Question E(6).*

Preadmission Screening and Annual Resident Review Level I Screening form *(continued)*

SECTION F: SUBMITTER INFORMATION/CERTIFICATION

In order to process the screen, the submitter must provide his/her name and address and sign below. If the individual has indications of serious MI (YES to D[5]) and/or MR or a related condition (YES to E[7]), submitters must also complete Section G (next page). If the individual has indications of neither, submitters do not have to complete Section G. The NF may not admit or retain individuals with indications of serious MI and/or MR or a related condition without further review by ODMH and/or ODMR/DD (OAC Rules 5101: 3-3-151 and 5101:3-3-152).

Last name: Brown
First name: Lisa
Street address: 456 Main Street
City: Springhouse
State: PA
Zip: 19477
Telephone Number: (214) 999-9900

I understand that this screening information may be relied upon in the payment of claims that will be from Federal and State funds, and that any willful falsification, or concealment of a material fact, may be prosecuted under Federal and State laws. I certify that to the best of my knowledge the foregoing information is true, accurate, and complete.

Signature: Lisa Brown
Title: RN
Date: 03-10-2017 (Month Day Year)
Employer: Sunnyside Care Facility

PASARR IDENTIFICATION SCREEN

SECTION G: MAILING ADDRESSES

Complete this section ONLY if the individual has indications of serious MI, MR, or a related condition.

(1) What address should be used for mailing results of the PASARR evaluation to the applicant/resident?

In care of:
Street address:
City: State: Zip: Telephone Number: (   )

(2) Please provide the following information about the individual's attending physician:

Last name: First name:
Street address:
City: State: Zip: Telephone Number: (   )

(continued)

Preadmission Screening and Annual Resident Review Level I Screening form *(continued)*

SECTION G: MAILING ADDRESSES *(continued)*

(3) If the individual has a legal representative, please provide the following information about the representative:

Last name		First name

Street address

City	State	Zip	Telephone Number ( )

(4) If the individual is an applicant to or resident of an NF, please provide the name and address of the NF:

Name of NF

Street address

City	State	Zip	First 4 letter of county

(5) If the individual is being discharged from a hospital, and the submitter is not employed by the discharging hospital, please provide the name of a contact person and the name and address of the discharging hospital:

Last name		First name

Discharging hospital

Street address

City	State	Zip	Telephone Number ( )

ADL checklists and flow sheets

ADL checklists and flow sheets are forms that are usually completed by a nursing assistant or a restorative nurse on each shift; then you review and sign them. These forms tell the health care team members about the patient's abilities, degree of independence, and special needs so they can determine the type of assistance the patient requires.

The following tools are examples of checklists and flow sheets that can be used to assess ADLs:

- Katz index
- Lawton scale
- Barthel index and scale.

Katz index

The Katz index ranks the patient's ability in six areas:

- bathing
- dressing
- toileting
- moving from wheelchair to bed and returning (transferring)
- continence
- feeding.

It describes the patient's functional level at a specific time and rates the patient's performance of each function on three levels: performing without help, needing some help, or having complete disability. (See *Rating ability to perform basic tasks*, page 270.)

Lawton scale

The Lawton scale of instrumental activities evaluates the patient's ability to perform complex personal care activities necessary for independent living. Activities include:

- using the telephone
- shopping
- preparing meals
- housekeeping
- doing laundry
- transportation
- taking medications
- managing finances.

Activities are rated as either 1 or 0 with the patient attaining the highest score of 8—indicating high function or independence. (See *Rating ability to perform complex tasks*, page 271.)

Barthel index and scale

The Barthel index and scale is used to evaluate:

- feeding
- moving from wheelchair to bed and returning (transferring)
- performing personal hygiene
- getting on and off the toilet
- bathing
- walking on a level surface or propelling a wheelchair
- going up and down stairs
- dressing and undressing
- maintaining bowel continence
- controlling the bladder.

Each item is scored according to the amount of assistance needed. Over time, results reveal improvement or decline. Another scale, the Barthel self-care rating scale, evaluates function in more detail. (See *Getting better or worse?* pages 273 to 275.)

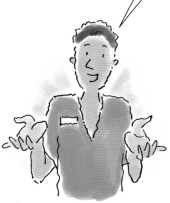

Assess your patient's ability to perform ADLs with the Katz index, Lawton scale, and Barthel index and scale.

(Text continues on page 272.)

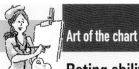

Rating ability to perform basic tasks

The Katz index, shown below, is used to assess six basic activities of daily living.

ACTIVITIES	INDEPENDENCE:	DEPENDENCE:
Points (1 or 0)	(1 POINT) NO supervision, direction, or personal assistance	(0 POINTS) WITH supervision, direction, personal assistance, or total care
BATHING Points: _0_	(1 POINT) Bathes self completely or needs help in bathing only a single part of the body such as the back, genital area, or disabled extremity.	(0 POINTS) Needs help with bathing more than one part of the body, getting in or out of the tub or shower. Requires total bathing.
DRESSING Points: _1_	(1 POINT) Gets clothes from closets and drawers and puts on clothes and outer garments complete with fasteners. May have help tying shoes.	(0 POINTS) Needs help with dressing self or needs to be completely dressed.
TOILETING Points: _0_	(1 POINT) Goes to toilet, gets on and off, arranges clothes, cleans genital area without help.	(0 POINTS) Needs help transferring to the toilet, cleaning self or uses bedpan or commode.
TRANSFERRING Points: _1_	(1 POINT) Moves in and out of bed or chair unassisted. Mechanical transferring aides are acceptable.	(0 POINTS) Needs help in moving from bed to chair or requires a complete transfer.
CONTINENCE Points: _0_	(1 POINT) Exercises complete self-control over urination and defecation.	(0 POINTS) Is partially or totally incontinent of bowel or bladder.
FEEDING Points: _1_	(1 POINT) Gets food from plate into mouth without help. Preparation of food may be done by another person.	(0 POINTS) Needs partial or total help with feeding or requires parenteral feeding.

TOTAL POINTS = _3_ 6 = High (patient independent) 0 = Low (patient very dependent)

Adapted with permission from the Gerontological Society of America. Katz, S., et al. "Progress in the Development of the Indexes of ADL," *The Gerontologist* 10(1):20-30, 1970.

Adapted version © 2000 by the Hartford Institute for Geriatric Nursing, College of Nursing, New York University. Used with permission.

Art of the chart

Rating ability to perform complex tasks

Patient Name: _____   Date: _____

Patient ID # _____

LAWTON - BRODY INSTRUMENTAL ACTIVITIES OF DAILY LIVING SCALE (I.A.D.L.)

Scoring: For each category, circle the item description that most closely resembles the client's highest functional level (either 0 or 1).

A. Ability to Use Telephone

1. Operates telephone on own initiative-looks up and dials numbers, etc.	1
2. Dials a few well-known numbers	1
3. Answers telephone but does not dial	1
4. Does not use telephone at all	0

B. Shopping

1. Takes care of all shopping needs independently	1
2. Shops independently for small purchases	0
3. Needs to be accompanied on any shopping trip	0
4. Completely unable to shop	0

C. Food Preparation

1. Plans, prepares and serves adequate meals independently	1
2. Prepares adequate meals if supplied with ingredients	1
3. Heats, serves and prepares meals, or prepares meals, or prepares meals but does not maintain adequate diet	1
4. Needs to have meals prepared and served	0

D. Housekeeping

1. Maintains house alone or with occasional assistance (e.g. "heavy work domestic help")	1
2. Performs light daily tasks such as dish washing, bed making	1
3. Performs light daily tasks but cannot maintain acceptable level of cleanliness	1
4. Needs help with all home maintenance tasks	1
5. Does not participate in any housekeeping tasks	0

E. Laundry

1. Does personal laundry completely	1
2. Launders small items-rinses stockings, etc.	1
3. All laundry must be done by others	0

F. Mode of Transportation

1. Travels independently on public transportation or drives own car	1
2. Arranges own travel via taxi, but does not otherwise use public transportation	1
3. Travels on public transportation when accompanied by another	1
4. Travel limited to taxi or automobile with assistance of another	0
5. Does not travel at all	0

(continued)

Rating ability to perform complex tasks *(continued)*

G. Responsibility for Own Medications		H. Ability to Handle Finances	
1. Is responsible for taking medication in correct dosages at correct time	1	1. Manages financial matters independently (budgets, writes checks, pays rent, bills, goes to bank), collects and keeps track of income	1
2. Takes responsibility if medication is prepared in advance in separate dosage	0	2. Manages day-to-day purchases, but needs help with banking, major purchases, etc.	1
3. Is not capable of dispensing own medication	0	3. Incapable of handling money	0
Score		**Score**	
		Total score _____	
A summary score ranges from 0 (low function, dependent) to 8 (high function, independent) for women and 0 through 5 for men to avoid potential gender bias.			

Source: Hartford Institute for Geriatric Nursing at New York University's College of Nursing. "Try this: Best Practices in Nursing Care to Older Adults," 2007. Available at: https://hign.org.

Care plans

Standards for care plans are developed by individual long-term care facilities. When a patient is admitted to a facility, an interim care plan is used until there's an interdisciplinary care conference regarding the patient. The interim care plan should be in place within 24 hours of admission. After the interim plan, a full care plan is developed for the patient. The interdisciplinary care plan should be completed within 7 days of the completion of the MDS. A documented review of the plan must be completed every 3 months or when the patient's status changes.

In long-term care settings, care plans usually evolve from an interdisciplinary approach to care, with contributions by the patient, members of the family, and other health care providers.

As always, base your care plan on the patient's health problems, nursing diagnoses, and expected treatment outcomes. Include measurable patient outcomes with reasonable time frames and specific interventions to achieve them.

Discharge and transfer forms

When the facility discharges a patient to home or to a hospital, you must document the reason for discharge, the patient's destination, the mode of transportation, and the person or staff member accompanying the patient, if appropriate.

(Text continues on page 275.)

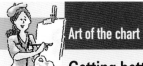

Art of the chart

Getting better or worse?

The Barthel index and scale (shown below) is used to assess the patient's ability to perform 10 activities of daily living, document findings for other health care team members, and reveal improvement or decline.

Patient Name: _Jack Boyd_

Evaluator: _Kate Roth, RN_

Date: _2/14/2017_

Activity	Score
FEEDING 0 = unable 5 = needs help cutting, spreading butter, etc., or requires modified diet 10 = independent	10
BATHING 0 = dependent 5 = independent (or in shower)	5
GROOMING 0 = needs to help with personal care 5 = independent face/hair/teeth/shaving (implements provided)	5
DRESSING 0 = dependent 5 = needs help but can do about half unaided 10 = independent (including buttons, zippers, laces, etc.)	5
BOWELS 0 = incontinent (or needs to be given enemas) 5 = occasional accident 10 = continent	5
BLADDER 0 = incontinent, or catheterized and unable to manage alone 5 = occasional accident 10 = continent	5
TOILET USE 0 = dependent 5 = needs some help, but can do some things alone 10 = independent (on and off, dressing, wiping)	5
TRANSFERS (BED TO CHAIR AND BACK) 0 = unable, no sitting balance 5 = major help (one or two people, physical), can sit 10 = minor help (verbal or physical) 15 = independent	10

(continued)

Getting better or worse? *(continued)*

MOBILITY (ON LEVEL SURFACES)   5
0 = immobile or <50 yards
5 = wheelchair independent, including corners, >50 yards
10 = walks with help of one person (verbal or physical) >50 yards
15 = independent (but may use any aid; for example, stick) >50 yards

STAIRS   5
0 = unable
5 = needs help (verbal, physical, carrying aid)
10 = independent

                                                        TOTAL SCORE
                                                        (0–100)
                                                        60

DEFINITION AND DISCUSSION OF SCORING
A patient scoring 100 is continent, feeds himself, dresses himself, gets up out of bed and chairs, bathes himself, walks at least a block, and can ascend and descend stairs. This does not mean that he is able to live alone: he may not be able to cook, keep house, and meet the public, but he is able to get along without attendant care.
Feeding
  10 = Independent. The patient can feed himself a meal from a tray or table when someone puts the food within his reach. He must put on an assistive device if this is needed, cut up the food, use salt and pepper, spread butter, etc. He must accomplish this in a reasonable time.
  5 = Some help is necessary (with cutting up food, etc., as listed above).
Bathing
  5 = Patient may use a bathtub or a shower, or take a complete sponge bath. He must be able to do all the steps involved, in whichever method is employed, without another person being present.
Grooming
  5 = Patient can wash hands and face, comb hair, clean teeth, and shave. He may use any kind of razor but he must put in blade or plug in razor without help as well as get it from drawer or cabinet. Female patient must put on her own makeup, if used, but need not braid or style hair.
Dressing
  10 = Patient is able to put on and remove and fasten all clothing (including any prescribed corset or braces), and tie shoe laces (unless patient requires adaptations for this). Such special clothing as suspenders, loafer shoes, or dresses that open down the front may be used when necessary.
  5 = Patient needs help in putting on and removing or fastening any clothing. He must do at least half the work himself and must accomplish this in a reasonable time. Female patient need not be scored on use of a brassiere or girdle unless these are prescribed garments.
Bowels
  10 = Patient is able to control his bowels without accidents. He can use a suppository or take an enema when necessary (as in spinal cord injury patients who have had bowel training).
  5 = Patient needs help in using a suppository or taking an enema or has occasional accidents.
Bladder
  10 = Patient is able to control his bladder day and night. Spinal cord injury patients who wear an external device and leg bag must put them on independently, clean and empty bag, and stay dry day and night.
  5 = Patient has occasional accidents or cannot wait for the bedpan or get to the toilet in time or needs help with an external device.
Toilet use
  10 = Patient is able to get on and off toilet, fasten and unfasten clothes, prevent soiling of clothes, and use toilet paper without help. He may use a wall bar or other stable object for support if needed. If he needs a bedpan instead of a toilet, he must be able to place it on a chair, empty it, and clean it.
  5 = Patient needs help to overcome imbalance, handle clothes, or use toilet paper.

Getting better or worse? *(continued)*

Transfers (bed to chair and back)

15 = Independent in all phases of this activity. Patient can safely approach the bed in his wheelchair, lock brakes, lift footrests, move safely to bed, lie down, come to a sitting position on the side of the bed, change the position of the wheelchair if necessary to transfer back into it safely, and return to the wheelchair.

10 = Either the patient needs some minimal help in some step of this activity, or needs to be reminded or supervised for safety in one or more parts of this activity.

5 = Patient can come to a sitting position without the help of a second person but needs to be lifted out of bed, or if he transfers with a great deal of help.

Mobility (on level surfaces)

15 = Patient can walk at least 50 yards without help or supervision. He may wear braces or prostheses and use crutches, a cane, or a walkerette but not a rolling walker. He must be able to lock and unlock braces if used, get the necessary mechanical aides into position for use, stand up and sit down, and dispose of them when he sits. (Putting on and taking off braces is scored under dressing.)

10 = Patient needs help or supervision in any of the above but can walk at least 50 yards with a little help.

5 = If a patient cannot ambulate but can propel a wheelchair independently, he must be able to go around corners, turn around, maneuver the chair to a table, bed, toilet, etc. He must be able to push a chair at least 50 yards. Do not score this item if the patient gets scored for walking.

Stairs

10 = Patient is able to go up and down a flight of stairs safely without help or supervision. He may and should use handrails, canes, or crutches when needed. He must be able to carry canes or crutches as he ascends or descends stairs.

5 = Patient needs help with or supervision of any one of the above items.

Adapted with permission from the Maryland State Medical Society. Mahoney, F.I., and Barthel, D.W. "Functional Evaluation: The Barthel Index," *Maryland State Medical Journal* 14:56-61, February 1965.

Guidelines drawn up by The Joint Commission emphasize the need to assess and summarize the patient's condition at transfer time. (See Transfer and personal belongings forms, page 276.)

> My patient is being discharged . . .

Other important data to include in this document are a list of prescribed medications, skin assessment findings, overall condition, the disposition of personal belongings, and teaching topics that you covered (such as diet, medications, skin care, and other areas).

Documentation guidelines

In long-term care facilities, consider the following points when updating your records:

- When writing nursing summaries, address specific patient problems noted in the care plan.

(Text continues on page 278.)

Art of the chart

Transfer and personal belongings forms

Patients in long-term care facilities may be admitted to the hospital, discharged to home, or transferred to other facilities. The forms below are used during this process.

1. PATIENT'S LAST NAME	FIRST NAME	MI	2. SEX	3. SOCIAL SECURITY NUMBER
Clark	*Robert*	*T*	*Male*	*144-44-4444*

4. PATIENT'S ADDRESS (Street, City, State, Zip Code)	5. DATE OF BIRTH	6. RELIGION
1 Wise street Springhouse, PA 19477	*2-8-28*	*unknown*

7. DATE OF THIS TRANSFER	8. FACILITY NAME AND ADDRESS TRANSFERRING TO	9. PHYSICIAN IN CHARGE AT TIME OF TRANSFER
2/28/2017	*Seniors Care Facility 22 Elderly Way Phila., PA*	*Dr. W. Nicholas* Will this physician care for patient after admission to new facility? ☐ YES ☒ NO

10. DATES OF STAY AT FACILITY TRANSFERRING FROM	11. PAYMENT SOURCE FOR CHARGES TO PATIENT
ADMISSION *1/14/2017* DISCHARGE *2/28/2017*	A. ☒ SELF OR FAMILY B. ☐ PRIVATE INSURANCE C. ☐ BLUE CROSS BLUE SHIELD D. ☐ EMPLOYER OR UNION E. ☐ PUBLIC AGENCY (Give name) F. ☐ OTHER (Explain)

12-A. NAME AND ADDRESS OF FACILITY TRANSFERRING FROM	12-B. NAMES AND ADDRESSES OF ALL HOSPITALS AND EXTENDED CARE FACILITIES FROM WHICH PATIENT WAS DISCHARGED IN PAST 60 DAYS.
Community Hospital 3000 Medical Way, Phila., PA	

13. CLINIC APPOINTMENT DATE TIME CLINIC APPOINTMENT CARD ATTACHED	14. DATE OF LAST PHYSICAL EXAMINATION *2/26/2017*

15. RELATIVE OR GUARDIAN:	Name	Address	Phone number
	Katherine Clark	*1 Wise Street Springhouse, PA 19477*	*1-215-999-9000*

16. DIAGNOSES AT TIME OF TRANSFER	EMPLOYMENT RELATED:
(a) Primary *Stroke* (b) Secondary *Type 1 diabetes*	☐ YES ☒ NO

VITALS AT TIME OF TRANSFER	ADVANCE DIRECTIVES ☐ YES ☒ NO ☐ COPY ATTACHED
T *98.6* P *68* R *20* B/P *140/82*	CODE STATUS *Full code*

CHECK ALL THAT APPLY

Disabilities
☐ Amputation
☑ Paralysis ⓁL side
☐ Contracture
☐ Pressure Ulcer

Impairments
☐ Mental
☑ Speech

☐ Hearing
☑ Vision
☐ Sensation

Incontinence
☑ Bladder
☑ Bowel
☑ Saliva

Activity Tolerance Limitations
☐ None
☑ Moderate
☐ Severe

Patient knows diagnosis?
☑ Yes
☐ No

Potential for Rehabilitation
☐ Good
☑ Fair
☐ Poor

IMPORTANT MEDICAL INFORMATION
(State allergies if any)
PCN

DIET, DRUGS, AND OTHER THERAPY at time of discharge
—Mechanical soft diet (2,000 cal)
—Megace 4 tabs Q6h
—Lasix 40 mg P.O. b.i.d.
—Aspirin 81mg P.O. daily
—Humulin 70/30 20 units daily in a.m. and at bedtime

(Physician, please sign below)

SUGGESTIONS FOR ACTIVE CARE

BED
Position in good body alignment and change position every *2* hrs.
Avoid *flat supine* position
Prone position *2* time/day as tolerated.

SITTING
4 hr *3* times/day

WEIGHT BEARING
☐ Full
☑ Partial
☐ None

on _____ Leg

EXERCISES
Range of motion *3* times/day.
to ⓁL *extremities* by
☐ patient ☐ nurse ☑ family
Stand *3* min. *2* times/day.

LOCOMOTION
Walk *unable* times/day.

SOCIAL ACTIVITIES
Encourage (☑ Group ☐ Individual)
activities (☑ within ☐ outside) home.
☐ Transportation: ☑ Ambulance
☐ Car ☐ Car for handicapped
☐ Bus

Signature of Physician or Nurse *John Brown, RN*   Date *2 / 28 / 2017*

Transfer and personal belongings forms *(continued)*

Any articles of clothing or other belongings left at the hospital will be held for 30 days after discharge. Items remaining after this period will be disposed of by the hospital.

		COMMENTS
Date: *2/28/2017*		
Initials: *CR*		
VALUABLES DESCRIBE		
Wallet:	✓	*1 brown leather wallet*
Money (Amount): *$25.00*	✓	*1–$20.00 bill 5 $ 1 bills*
Watch:		
Jewelry:		
Glasses/Contacts: *Glasses*	✓	*Wire rim–gold*
Hearing Aids:		
Dentures:	✓	
Partial		
Complete	✓	*Container labeled*
Keys		
ARTICLE DESCRIBE		
Ambulatory Aids:		
Cane, Walker, Etc.		
Bedclothes	✓	*1 pair plaid pajamas*
Belt		
Dress		
Outer Wear		
Pants		
Pocketbook		
Shirt		
Shoes		
Sweater		
Undergarments		
Other		

All belongings were sent home with patient's family: YES   (NO)

Patient's Signature ___*Bob Park*___

Witnessed by Hospital Personnel ___*Mary Jones, RN*___

- When writing progress notes, confirm that the patient's progress is being evaluated and reevaluated in relation to the goals or outcomes in the care plan. If goals aren't met, address this. Also, describe and document additional actions.
- Record transfers and discharges according to facility protocol.
- Document changes in the patient's condition, and report them to the practitioner and the family within 24 hours.
- Document follow-up interventions or other measures taken in response to a change in the patient's condition.
- Keep a record of visits from family or friends and of phone calls about the patient. State or federal regulators may fine your facility if these aren't documented.
- If an incident occurs, such as a fall or a treatment error, fill out an incident report and write follow-up notes for at least 48 hours after the incident (or follow your facility's policy).
- During the patient's first week of residence, keep detailed records on each shift.
- Flag a new patient by putting a red dot on the chart, bed, or door or by using a similar system so that all staff members are aware of the new resident and become familiar with the patient. (Remember, however, to be sensitive to each patient's need for confidentiality and dignity.)
- Keep reimbursement in mind when documenting. For a facility to qualify for payment, its records must clearly reflect the level of care given to the patient.
- Make sure that your records accurately reflect skilled services the patient receives.
- Always record a practitioner's verbal and telephone orders, and have the practitioner countersign them within 48 hours.
- Document visits by the practitioner to the patient. Generally accepted standards require one visit after admission, another after the first 30 days, and at least one every 60 days thereafter. However, the resident's condition ultimately guides the frequency of practitioner's visits.

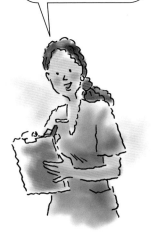

... that means I need to fill out another form.

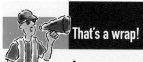

That's a wrap!

Long-term care documentation review

The basics
• Documentation isn't done as often for patients in long-term care.
• It can be extensive because of the long government forms involved.

Regulatory agencies
• *Medicare* provides reimbursement for patients requiring skilled care if minimum daily documentation is done to prove need.
• *Medicaid* provides reimbursement for patients who receive skilled care. To ensure reimbursement, document care once per day.
• The *Centers for Medicare & Medicaid Services (CMS)* requires staff members of long-term care facilities to complete the *Minimum Data Set (MDS)*, review the patient's status every 3 months, and perform a comprehensive reassessment annually.
• *Omnibus Budget Reconciliation Act (OBRA)* was enacted by Congress in 1987 to protect the rights of patients. Regulations include specifics for patient assessments and care plans.
• The Joint Commission accredits long-term care facilities.

Forms used in long-term care
• MDS is a multidisciplinary form that's mandated by OBRA and must be completed for every long-term care patient.
• *Preadmission Screening and Annual Resident Review (PASARR)* documents complete assessment of the patient's mental status.
• The *initial assessment form* is similar to the initial assessment form used in other settings but places greater emphasis on activity, hearing and vision, bowel and bladder control, communication, safety, assistive devices, family relationships, and transition.
• The *nursing summary* must be completed once per month and describes the patient's ability to perform activities of daily living (ADLs), nutrition and hydration status, safety measures, treatments, and problems adjusting to the long-term care facility.
• *ADL checklists and flow sheets* indicate the patient's abilities, degree of independence, and special needs to determine the type of assistance the patient requires.
• *Care plans* usually evolve from an interdisciplinary approach to care and should always be based on the patient's health problems, nursing diagnoses, and expected outcomes.
• *Discharge and transfer forms* must include the reason for discharge as well as the patient's destination and mode of transportation.

Documentation guidelines
• In nursing summaries, address patient problems.
• In progress notes, evaluate progress.
• Record transfers and discharges.
• Document changes in the patient's condition and follow-up information.
• Keep a record of family and friend visits and phone calls.
• If an incident occurs, fill out an incident report and write follow-up notes for 48 hours.
• Keep detailed records during the patient's first week.
• Make sure records clearly reflect the level of care for reimbursement purposes.
• Record the practitioner's verbal and telephone orders, and have them signed within 48 hours.
• Document visits by the practitioner.

Suggested references

Centers for Medicare & Medicaid Services. "Long-Term Care Facility Resident
  Assessment Instrument 3.0 User's Manual. Version 1.15," 2017. Available:
  https://downloads.cms.gov/files/MDS-30-RAI-Manual-v115-October
  -2017.pdf.

Congress.gov. "H.R. 3545: Omnibus Budget Reconciliation Act of 1987," n.d. Available:
  https://www.congress.gov/bill/100th-congress/house-bill/3545.

Federal Interagency Forum on Aging-Related Statistics. "Older Americans Key Indicators
  of Well-being," 2016. Available: https://agingstats.gov/docs/LatestReport
  /Older-Americans-2016-Key-Indicators-of-WellBeing.pdf.

Graf, C. "The Lawton Instrumental Activities of Daily Living (IADL) scale," 2013.
  Available: https://consultgeri.org/try-this/general-assessment/issue-23.pdf.

He, W., et al. "An Aging World: 2015. International Population Reports," 2015. Available:
  https://www.census.gov/content/dam/Census/library/publications/2016
  /demo/p95-16-1.pdf.

Medicaid.gov. "Preadmission Screening and Resident Review," n.d. Available:
  https://www.medicaid.gov/medicaid/ltss/institutional/pasrr/index.html.

PASRR Technical Assistance Center. "PASRR in Plain English," 2016. Available:
  http://www.pasrrassist.org/resources/federal-regulations/pasrr-plain-english.

United States Census. "Quick Facts," 2016. Available: https://www.census.gov
  /quickfacts/fact/table/US/PST045216#viewtop.

Appendices and index

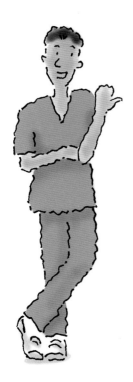

Accountability: obligation to accept responsibility for or account for one's actions

Accreditation: official recognition from a professional or government organization that a health care facility meets relevant standards

Advance directive: document used as a guideline for life-sustaining medical care of a patient with an advanced disease or disability, who's no longer able to communicate wishes regarding end-of-life care; includes living wills and durable powers of attorney for health care

Bar code technology: utilization of a bar code system that matches patient information to interventions, such as medication and blood administration to increase safety and decrease errors

Barthel index and scale: functional assessment tool used to evaluate an older patient's overall well-being and self-care abilities; evaluates the ability to perform 10 self-care activities

Care pathway: documentation tool used in managed care and case management in which a time line is defined for the patient's condition and for the achievement of expected outcomes; used by caregivers to determine on any given day where the patient should be on progressing toward optimal health

Care plan: a listing of the patient's identified problems, needs, and measurable goals with instructions for achieving the goals; used to direct care

Case management: model for management of health care facilities in which one professional—usually a nurse or a social worker—assumes responsibility for coordinating care so that patients move through the health care system in the shortest time and at the lowest possible cost

Centers for Medicare & Medicaid Services (CMS): a branch of the U.S. Department of Health and Human Services, CMS regulates compliance with federal Medicare and Medicaid standards; CMS regulations are usually enforced at the state level.

Charting by exception (CBE): documentation system that departs from traditional systems by requiring documentation of only significant or abnormal findings

Commission on Accreditation of Rehabilitation Facilities (CARF): independent, nonprofit organization that provides accreditation to qualifying rehabilitation facilities worldwide

Community Health Accreditation Partner (CHAP): organization that partners with home health care providers to assist with and provide accreditation

Contraband: any item that's prohibited from being in the patient's possession while residing in a facility

Database: subjective and objective patient information collected during your initial assessment of the patient; includes information obtained by taking your patient's health history, performing a physical examination, and analyzing laboratory test results

Diagnosis-related group (DRG): system of classifying or grouping patients according to medical diagnosis for purposes of reimbursement of hospitalization costs under Medicare

Discharge summary: documentation that reflects the patient's condition from admission to discharge completed when the patient is ready to leave a facility

Do-not-resuscitate (DNR) orders: instructions not to attempt to resuscitate a patient in cardiac or respiratory arrest

Durable power of attorney for health care: legal document whereby a patient authorizes another person to make medical decisions should the patient becomes incompetent to do so

Electronic health record (EHR): computerized data system designed to retain patient information more efficiently and to transfer patient information easily between health care settings

Electronic medication administration record (eMAR): computerized system of medication administration documentation; usually utilizes bar code technology

Flow sheet: documentation tool that highlights specific patient information according to preestablished parameters of nursing care

FOCUS (F-DAR) documentation: documentation system that uses assessment data, first to evaluate patient-centered topics (or foci of concern) and then to document precisely and concisely

Harassment: verbal or physical conduct that denigrates or shows hostility or aversion toward another individual based on race, culture, color, religion, gender, sexual orientation, national origin, age, culture, or disability

Health history: summary of a patient's health status that includes physiologic, psychological, cultural, and psychosocial data

Hostile advances: behavior that is threatening in nature toward another person

Incident report: formal written report that informs facility administrators (and the facility's insurance company) about an incident and that serves as a contemporary factual statement in the event of a lawsuit

Informed consent: permission obtained from a patient to perform a specific test or procedure after the patient has been fully informed about the test or procedure, including the risks and benefits

Interventions: nursing actions taken to meet a patient's health care needs; should reflect nurse's agreement with the patient on how to meet defined goals or expected outcomes

Kardex: document that provides a quick overview of basic patient care information; not a part of the patient's medical record

Katz index: assessment tool used to evaluate a patient's ability to perform the basic functions of bathing, dressing, toileting, transferring, continence, and feeding

Lawton scale: assessment tool used to evaluate a patient's ability to perform relatively complex tasks, such as using a telephone, cooking, managing finances, and taking medications

Learning outcomes: outcomes developed as part of a patient-teaching plan that identify what a patient needs to learn, how you'll provide that teaching, and how you'll evaluate what the patient has learned

Living will: witnessed document indicating a patient's wishes for end-of-life care; applies to decisions that will be made after a terminally ill patient is incompetent and has no reasonable possibility of recovery

Medication reconciliation: review of home medications for accuracy and current use that occurs on admission to a facility as well as prior to transfer or discharge

Minimum Data Set (MDS): standardized assessment tool that must be filled out for every patient admitted to a long-term care facility as mandated by the federal government (OBRA)

Multidisciplinary team: health care workers from various departments (disciplines) who participate in a patient's care

NANDA International (NANDA-I): organization responsible for developing and categorizing nursing diagnoses and examining applications of nursing diagnoses in clinical practice, education, and research

Narrative documentation system: method of documentation utilizing a written note to record information regarding the patient

National Patient Safety Goals (NPSGs): standards set by the Joint Commission to increase patient safety and decrease medical errors

Nurse practice act: state laws that designate a nurse's scope of practice in that particular state

Nursing diagnosis: clinical judgment made by a nurse regarding a patient's actual or potential health problems or life processes; describes a patient problem that the nurse can address; may apply to families and communities as well as individual patients

Nursing information systems (NISs): software programs that allow the nurse to record assessment, interventions, and outcomes in the electronic health record; can be customized to conform to facilities needs

Nursing Minimum Data Set (NMDS): a means of standardizing nursing information; contains three categories of information—nursing care, patient demographics, and service elements

Nursing Outcomes Classification (NOC): classification systems that provides standardization of the terminology and criteria related to patient outcomes

Nursing process: systematic approach to identifying a patient's problems and identifying nursing interventions to address them; steps include assessing the patient's problems, forming a diagnostic statement, identifying expected outcomes, creating a plan to achieve expected outcomes and solve the patient's problems, implementing the plan or assigning others to implement it, and evaluating the plan's effectiveness

Occurrence reporting: reporting by practitioners, nurses, or other staff of unusual or dangerous incidents, either when they're observed or shortly after; also called *incident reporting*

Occurrence screening: identification of adverse events through a review of medical records

Omnibus Budget Reconciliation Act (OBRA): law enacted in 1987 establishing specific requirements for long-term facilities and home-health agencies to protect the rights of patients

Outcome and Assessment Information Set (OASIS): assessment of all Medicare and Medicaid patients older than age 18 years, excluding women receiving maternal–child services who are receiving skilled services

Outcome criteria: standards by which measurable goals, or outcomes, are objectively evaluated

Outcome documentation: documentation that focuses on patient behaviors and responses to nursing care; documents the patient's condition in relation to predetermined outcomes included in the care plan

Patient Self-Determination Act: law that requires health care facilities to provide information about the patient's right to choose and refuse treatment

Patient-teaching plan: an organized plan which identifies learning needs for the patient; pinpoints how teaching will be accomplished and criteria for evaluating how well the patient learns

Physician Orders for Life-Sustaining Treatment (POLST): legal document that contains physician orders for end-of-life treatment as agreed upon by the patient; must be honored by facilities when presented

Preadmission Screening and Annual Resident Review (PASARR): evaluation to assess the mental status of a patient before admission to a long-term care facility to determine if the facility is the most appropriate to provide needed care; required for Medicare or Medicaid reimbursement

Problem-oriented medical record (POMR): method of organizing the medical record; consists of baseline data, a problem list, and a care plan for each problem

Quality management: commitment on the part of a health care facility or several health disciplines to work together to achieve an optimal degree of excellence in the services rendered to every patient (state regulatory and accrediting agencies may require health care facilities to regularly monitor, evaluate, and seek ways to improve the quality of care)

Rapid response team: team of skilled health care workers who are called to assess a hospitalized patient (on non-intensive care units) who has signs of deterioration in order to prevent a cardiac or respiratory arrest

Resident assessment instrument (RAI): form required by federal mandate for use in long-term care facilities that identifies the patient's primary problems and care needs and documents the existence of a care plan

Risk management: identification, analysis, evaluation, and elimination or reduction of risks to patients, visitors, or employees; involves loss prevention and control and the handling of all incidents, claims, and other insurance- and litigation-related tasks

Sexual harassment: offensive, unwelcome, or unwanted conduct of a sexual nature, which may include nonverbal, verbal, or physical behavior

SOAP documentation: structured method of documentation in which data are organized into four categories: Subjective, Objective, Assessment, and Planning

SOAPIE documentation: structured method of documentation in which data are organized into six categories: Subjective, Objective, Assessment, Planning, Implementation, and Evaluation

SOAPIER documentation: structured method of documentation in which data are organized into seven categories: Subjective, Objective, Assessment, Planning, Implementation, Evaluation, and Revision

The Joint Commission: private, nongovernmental agency that establishes guidelines for the operation of hospitals and other health care facilities, conducts accreditation programs and surveys, and encourages the attainment of high standards of institutional medical care; members include representatives from the American Medical Association, American College of Physicians, and American College of Surgeons

Transfusion administration record: documentation tool utilized for the administration of blood products

Utilization review: program initiated by reimbursing agents to maintain control over health care providers that may focus on length of stay, treatment regimen, validation of tests and procedures, and verification of the use of medical supplies and equipment

Index

Note: i refers to an illustration; t refers to a table.

Note: i refers to an illustration; t refers to a table.

Note: i refers to an illustration; t refers to a table.

Note: i refers to an illustration; t refers to a table.

Note: i refers to an illustration; t refers to a table.

Note: i refers to an illustration; t refers to a table.